0 POINT WEIGHT LOSS COOKBOOK

Ultimate Guide to Effortless and Guilt-Free Recipes for Sustainable Weight Loss.

Includes 28-Day Meal Plan and Tips for a Healthier Lifestyle

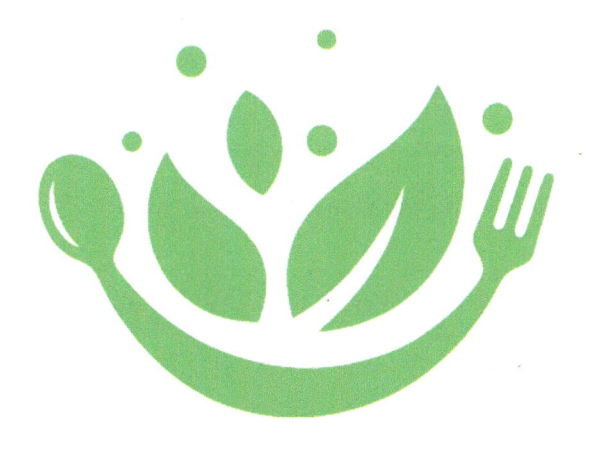

Adam Blanton

Cover and Layout: thebookslab.com

Copyright © 2024 [Adam Blanton]

All rights reserved. No part of this guide may be reproduced in any form without permission in writing from the publisher except in the case of brief quotations embodied in critical articles or reviews.

Legal & Disclaimer

The information contained in this book and its contents is not designed to replace or take the place of any form of medical or professional advice; and is not meant to replace the need for independent medical, financial, legal or other professional advice or services, as may be required.

You agree to accept all risks of using the information presented inside this book.

You agree that by continuing to read this book, where appropriate and/or necessary, you shall consult a professional (including but not limited to your doctor, or such other advisor as needed) before using any of the suggested remedies, techniques, or information in this book.

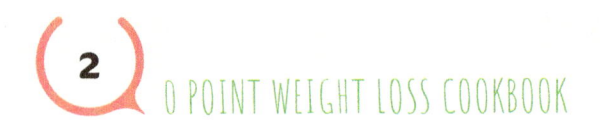

Contents

Introduction: The Concept of "0 Points" 5
    Welcome to the World of Stress-Free Weight Loss 5
    What Does "0 Points" Mean? 5
    Why This Approach Works 5

Chapter 1: Fundamental Principles of the "0 Points" Diet 6
    A New Approach to Weight Loss 6
    The Philosophy Behind "0 Points" Foods 6
    Ease of Long-Term Adherence 6
    The Importance of Hydration and Low-Calorie Foods 7
    Managing Special Occasions and Eating Out 7
    Integrating Exercise Routines with the "0 Points" Diet 7
    Setting Yourself Up for Success 7

Chapter 2: "0 Points" Foods. What and Why 8
    Why Include "0 Points" Foods in Your Diet? 8
    How to Integrate "0 Points" Foods into Every Meal 8
    Detailed List of "0 Points" Foods 9
    How "0 Points" Foods Promote Satiety Without Adding Excess Calories 10
    Tips on How to Integrate "0 Points" Foods into Daily Diets 10

Chapter 3: Meal Planning and Portion Management 11
    Planning Meals with "0 Points" Foods 11
    Weekly Meal Plan Examples 12
    Grocery Shopping Tips 12
    Adjustments for Special Occasions 12

Chapter 4: Overcoming Common Challenges — 14
- Common Challenges in the "0 Points" Diet — 14
- Managing Hunger — 14
- Variety in the Diet — 14
- Tips for Maintaining Motivation and Long-Term Adherence to the Diet Plan — 15

Chapter 5: Integrating Physical Activity — 16
- The Importance of Exercise in Combination with the "0 Points" Diet — 16
- Tips for Incorporating Physical Activity into Your Daily Routine, Regardless of Fitness Level — 16

Chapter 6: Introduction to Recipes — 18
- Preparing for Recipes — 18
- Structure of Recipes — 18
- Kitchen Tips — 18

Chapter 7: Recipes — 20
- Breakfasts — 21
- Lunches — 29
- Snacks — 37
- Dinners — 45
- Desserts — 53
- Beverages and Smoothies — 59

28-Day Meal Plan — 65

Measurement Conversions — 68

Conclusion — 70

Recipe Index — 72

BONUS — 74

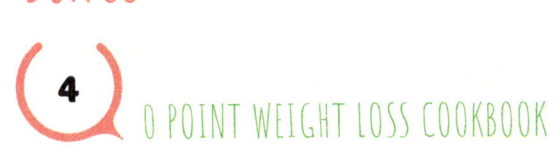

Introduction: The Concept of "0 Points"

Welcome to the World of Stress-Free Weight Loss

Losing weight can often seem like a daunting task filled with restrictions and complications. However, the concept of "0 points" was born to simplify your journey towards a healthier life. In this book, you will discover how to integrate delicious and nutritious foods into your daily diet without having to count every single calorie. My mission is to help you achieve your weight loss goals sustainably, giving you the freedom to enjoy food without guilt.

What Does "0 Points" Mean?

The "0 points" diet is based on a simple principle: there are foods you can consume freely without the need to weigh, measure, or count their points or calories. These foods have been selected for their high nutritional density and low-calorie content. They are rich in fiber, protein, and other essential nutrients that help you feel fuller longer and boost your metabolism. By eating these foods, you can reduce your daily calorie intake without compromising on taste or variety in your diet.

Why This Approach Works

Many diet programs fail because they are too restrictive or difficult to follow in the long term. The "0 points" diet offers a more flexible and manageable approach. Without the worry of exceeding a daily points or calorie limit, you can focus on what really matters: nourishing your body and enjoying meals. This method not only makes it easier to maintain weight loss but also promotes a positive change in attitude towards food and eating. Through this guide, you will learn how to make smart food choices that can transform your body and overall well-being.

By the way, at the end of this book, **you will find a BONUS** that you can download for free. It will help you expand and deepen the knowledge you learned with this book! I would be very happy if you downloaded it and at the same time left a review on amazon, **I would appreciate it very much!**

Chapter 1: Fundamental Principles of the "0 Points" Diet

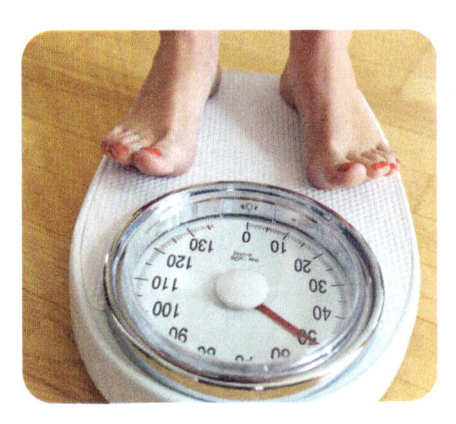

A New Approach to Weight Loss

When we think about weight loss, we often imagine restrictive and complex diets that require constant calorie counting. The "0 points" diet breaks away from this traditional pattern by offering a **liberating and sustainable approach to wellness**. This method not only eliminates the need to measure every bite but allows you to focus on listening to your body and fulfilling its true nutritional needs.

The Philosophy Behind "0 Points" Foods

At the heart of the "0 points" diet is a **careful selection of foods** that you can consume freely. These foods, chosen for their high nutrient content and low-calorie intake, include fresh fruits, non-starchy vegetables, and lean proteins. The goal is to encourage the consumption of foods that intensively nourish without significantly contributing to the daily calorie count. This selection helps maintain satiety, reduce cravings, and support an active metabolism.

Adopting the "0 points" diet is not only an effective strategy for weight loss but also promotes overall health improvement. **"0 points" foods are rich in fiber, vitamins, and essential minerals** that contribute to digestive health, improve heart function, and strengthen the immune system. By integrating these foods into your daily diet, you will not only work towards your weight goals but also elevate the overall quality of your nutrition and lifestyle.

Ease of Long-Term Adherence

One of the most challenging aspects of many diets is maintaining consistency and motivation in the long term. The "0 points" diet addresses this challenge by **eliminating the need to count calories or points**. This simplification transforms the weight loss process from a burdensome task to a sustainable habit. Moreover, the freedom to consume a variety of "0 points" foods reduces the risk of frustration and abandonment that often occurs with more restrictive diets.

Integrating "0 points" foods into your daily diet is simple and highly customizable. Whether you are preparing a quick lunch or planning a family dinner, you can build rich and satisfying dishes around these foods. Examples include fruit smoothies, rich salads, vegetable stews, and dishes based on lean proteins like chicken or fish. **The key is creativity in meal preparation, experimenting with herbs and spices** to enhance flavors without adding calories.

To get the most out of the "0 points" diet, it is important to **balance your meals with a variety of "0 points" foods** to ensure complete nutritional intake. It is also essential to listen to your body and adjust portions according to your actual energy needs, especially if you are physically active. Alongside "0 points" foods, consider including moderate portions of other nutrient-rich foods that have a caloric cost, such as whole grains and healthy fats, to maintain balance and promote optimal health.

The Importance of Hydration and Low-Calorie Foods

An often overlooked aspect of diets is the importance of hydration. Water plays a crucial role in maintaining health and regulating metabolism. In the "0 points" diet, I strongly encourage the consumption of ample liquids, especially water, unsweetened teas, and vegetable broths, which can help you feel full and satisfied. These liquids support digestion and can increase the sense of satiety, reducing the likelihood of consuming high-calorie foods between meals.

Managing Special Occasions and Eating Out

A common challenge in diets is how to maintain dietary commitments during social events or meals at restaurants. In the "0 points" diet, I will provide you with strategies to navigate these situations without stress. You will learn to choose smart food options that respect the principles of the diet even when you are not at home. This includes tips on how to order at restaurants, which foods to prioritize at buffets, and how to handle special occasions without deviating from your weight loss path.

Integrating Exercise Routines with the "0 Points" Diet

Exercise is an essential complement to any weight loss plan. Not only does it help burn calories, but it also improves mental and physical health. In the "0 points" diet, we will discuss how to integrate physical activities that enhance your weight loss efforts without overloading your schedule. From daily walks to high-intensity interval training, there are options suitable for every fitness level and lifestyle.

Setting Yourself Up for Success

In concluding this chapter, my goal has been to provide you with the knowledge and tools necessary to successfully start your journey on the "0 points" diet. Remember, the path to sustainable weight loss and optimal health is not always linear, but with the right tools and an open mindset, you can make this journey both enjoyable and effective.

Chapter 2: "0 Points" Foods. What and Why

The idea of "0 points" foods is at the core of the diet I promote. These foods have been chosen not only for their low caloric content but especially for their high content of essential nutrients. In this chapter, we will explore what makes these foods special and why they can be consumed without restrictions, facilitating weight loss and maintaining a balanced diet.

"0 points" foods are rich in vital components such as fiber, protein, vitamins, and minerals but low in calories. This makes them ideal for inclusion in a low-calorie diet. Foods like fresh fruits and vegetables, legumes, skinless chicken breast, and fish are all examples of food choices you can freely enjoy. Each food group offers specific benefits: vegetables provide essential fibers and micronutrients; fruits are a great source of natural antioxidants; and lean proteins support the building and maintenance of muscle mass.

Why Include "0 Points" Foods in Your Diet?

Including "0 points" foods in your daily diet has numerous benefits. **First, they help control total caloric intake without sacrificing the volume or quality of meals.** This is crucial for those looking to lose weight without feeling deprived or hungry. Additionally, these foods can improve overall health and prevent chronic diseases thanks to their richness in nutrients and antioxidants. The variety of "0 points" foods also allows you to maintain a varied and interesting diet, avoiding the monotony that often accompanies other diets.

Incorporating a wide range of "0 points" foods is not only a strategy to maintain interest in your diet but is also essential to achieve a complete nutritional profile. Diversifying your diet with a variety of fruits, vegetables, legumes, and lean proteins ensures that you receive a full range of essential amino acids, vitamins, minerals, and other phytonutrients that support the immune system, improve skin health, and optimize digestive function.

How to Integrate "0 Points" Foods into Every Meal

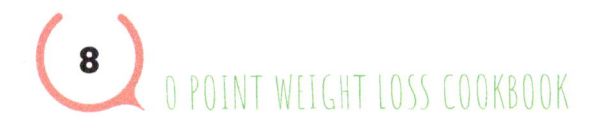

To make the most of "0 points" foods, it is useful to consider how they can be integrated into every meal. For breakfast, for example, you could add fresh fruit and spinach to a protein smoothie. For lunch, a rich salad with various types of vegetables and a source of lean protein can be a satisfying and nutritious meal. Dinner might include a generous portion of steamed or grilled vegetables and baked fish. Even snacks can be enriched with "0 points" foods, such as raw vegetable sticks or a small bowl of fresh berries.

"0 points" foods are particularly useful in this context because they allow for larger quantities of food that help you feel full longer. Incorporating these foods regularly into your eating routines can help control appetite and prevent overeating that often leads to weight gain.

Detailed List of "0 Points" Foods

Now let's see what versatile and nutritious "0 points" foods can be consumed in abundance. Here's a list categorized for ease:

Vegetables (non-starchy)

- Lettuce (all types)
- Spinach
- Kale
- Broccoli
- Cauliflower
- Zucchini
- Bell peppers
- Asparagus
- Tomatoes
- Cucumbers
- Mushrooms
- Carrots
- Celery
- Fennel
- Cabbage

Fruits

- Apples
- Oranges
- Strawberries
- Raspberries
- Melon
- Grapefruit
- Peaches
- Pears
- Kiwi
- Watermelon
- Blueberries
- Plums

Lean Proteins

- Skinless chicken breast
- Lean turkey
- Lean fish (such as cod, sole, tilapia)
- Eggs
- Legumes (lentils, various beans, chickpeas)
- Fat-free plain Greek yogurt
- Tofu
- Tempeh

Broths

- Vegetable broth (no added fats)
- Fat-free chicken broth
- Fat-free beef broth

Condiments

- Vinegar (all types except sweetened)

- Lemon and lime
- Fresh or dried herbs and spices (no added sugars or fats)
- Low-sodium soy sauce
- Mustard

Beverages

- Water (still or sparkling)
- Green, black, or herbal tea (no added sugars)
- Coffee (no added sugars or cream)

This detailed list provides a wide variety to facilitate meal planning and encourage a more varied and balanced diet. **Using these foods, you can create virtually endless combinations for tasty and satisfying meals.**

How "0 Points" Foods Promote Satiety Without Adding Excess Calories

One of the keys to the success of the "0 points" diet is the ability of these foods to promote satiety while being low in calories. **Foods rich in fiber and protein, such as legumes, raw vegetables, and lean proteins, take longer to chew and digest.** This slower process helps you feel full longer, reducing the need to eat frequently or in large quantities. Additionally, the presence of soluble fibers in legumes and fruit can slow the absorption of sugars into the bloodstream, stabilizing glucose levels and contributing to prolonged feelings of fullness. The combination of these factors makes "0 points" foods powerful tools for weight control and appetite management.

Tips on How to Integrate "0 Points" Foods into Daily Diets

Integrating "0 points" foods into your daily diet can be simple and creative. Here are some practical suggestions:

- **Start the Day with a Fiber-Rich Breakfast:** Incorporate fruits and vegetables into smoothies or whole grains to start the day with energy.

- **Smart Snacks:** Use raw vegetables like carrots, cucumbers, or bell peppers with hummus or Greek yogurt for a snack that satisfies without weighing you down.

- **Balanced Main Meals:** Ensure that each meal contains a good portion of lean proteins and plenty of vegetables. For example, a bowl of salad with grilled chicken breast and a variety of colorful vegetables can be both satisfying and nutritious.

- **Experiment with Herbs and Spices:** To keep your dishes interesting and tasty, explore the use of different herbs and spices. This not only adds variety to your dishes but also potential health benefits without added calories.

- **Meal Preparation:** Dedicate some time to meal preparation for the week to simplify the integration of "0 points" foods. Prepare salads, soups, or stews in advance that can be easily reheated and served.

Using these tips, you can easily integrate "0 points" foods into your diet, making it richer and more varied while reducing the stress caused by more stringent diets.

Chapter 3: Meal Planning and Portion Management

Planning Meals with "0 Points" Foods

Effective meal planning is a fundamental pillar for the long-term success of any diet, especially when using "0 points" foods. Organizing meals around these foods not only ensures that your caloric intake remains low but also that your body receives optimal nutrition.

- **Vary Your Foods:** Variety not only prevents food boredom but also ensures that you receive a broad spectrum of essential nutrients. Experiment with different types of vegetables and lean proteins throughout the week to keep your meals interesting and nutritious.
- **Preparation in Advance:** Dedicating a few hours to meal preparation over the weekend can transform your weekly routine. Cook large batches of vegetables, grill several portions of proteins, and store everything in separate containers in the fridge. This not only saves time during the week but also helps you resist the temptation to deviate from your diet.
- **Useful Tools:** Use tools like meal planning apps or portion containers that can help you control quantities while diversifying foods. These resources can simplify the planning process and help you stay organized.

Eating "0 points" foods does not mean you can consume unlimited quantities. It is essential to understand and manage portions to ensure a balanced diet and avoid overeating, even if the foods are low in calories.

- **Using Measuring Tools:** For proteins and carbohydrates not classified as "0 points," using kitchen scales or measuring cups can help ensure that portions remain appropriate. Even for "0 points" foods, consider using similar tools initially to get an idea of portion sizes. Once you have a habit of understanding quantities, you can abandon scales and measuring cups.
- **Listening to Body Signals:** Cultivate the habit of listening carefully to your body. Learn to recognize when you are genuinely hungry and when you are simply bored or stressed. Taking a pause before serving yourself a second plate can give you time to assess if you are truly still hungry.
- **Food Education:** Understanding the nutritional value of foods can play a crucial role in portion management. Educating yourself on what and how much to eat can transform your approach to food, making you more aware of your dietary choices and their impacts on your body.

Weekly Meal Plan Examples

Here is a small example of a meal plan that includes two days to give you a quick idea of how to alternate and balance meals:

Monday:

- **Breakfast:** Spinach and Berry Smoothie with a spoonful of Greek yogurt.
- **Lunch:** Large salad with lettuce, tomatoes, cucumbers, grilled chicken breast.
- **Dinner:** Baked salmon with a mix of grilled vegetables (peppers, zucchini, asparagus).
- **Snacks:** Carrot and cucumber sticks with hummus.

Tuesday:

- **Breakfast:** Omelette with spinach, tomatoes, and mushrooms.
- **Lunch:** Lentil soup and a small green salad.
- **Dinner:** Baked turkey breast with steamed cauliflower and broccoli.
- **Snacks:** Sliced apple with a pinch of cinnamon.

These examples are just a taste (if you allow me the pun) of what you will find at the end of this book. To further support you on your journey to a healthier and more active life, I have included a complete 28-day meal plan based on the same nutritional principles discussed in this chapter.

This detailed plan will provide you with daily guidance, helping you to vary meals while maintaining a balanced caloric intake and enjoying the freedom that "0 points" foods can offer. I hope this helps you see the versatility and sustainability of the "0 points" diet, making it not just a diet but a lifestyle.

Grocery Shopping Tips

Grocery shopping can be one of the most critical aspects of your diet's success. Here are some tips to help you navigate the supermarket effectively and stay true to your health goals:

Plan Ahead: Before going to the supermarket, prepare a detailed shopping list based on your weekly meal plan. This helps avoid impulsive purchases of foods not in line with the "0 points" diet.

Shop on a Full Stomach: Shopping when you are satiated can reduce the temptation to buy snacks or foods that are not part of your meal plan.

Focus on the Perimeter of the Supermarket: Generally, fresh foods like fruits, vegetables, and lean proteins are found on the edges of the supermarket, while more processed and less healthy foods are located in the central aisles.

Adjustments for Special Occasions

Participating in social events or celebrating holidays does not mean you have to abandon your meal plan. Here's how you can stay on track even during special occasions:

Offer to Bring a Dish: When attending a lunch or dinner, offer to bring a dish that aligns with your diet. This ensures that there is at least one healthy option available for you.

Choose Wisely: If eating out, look for menu options that are close to "0 points" foods or ask for modifications to dishes to make them more compliant with your diet.

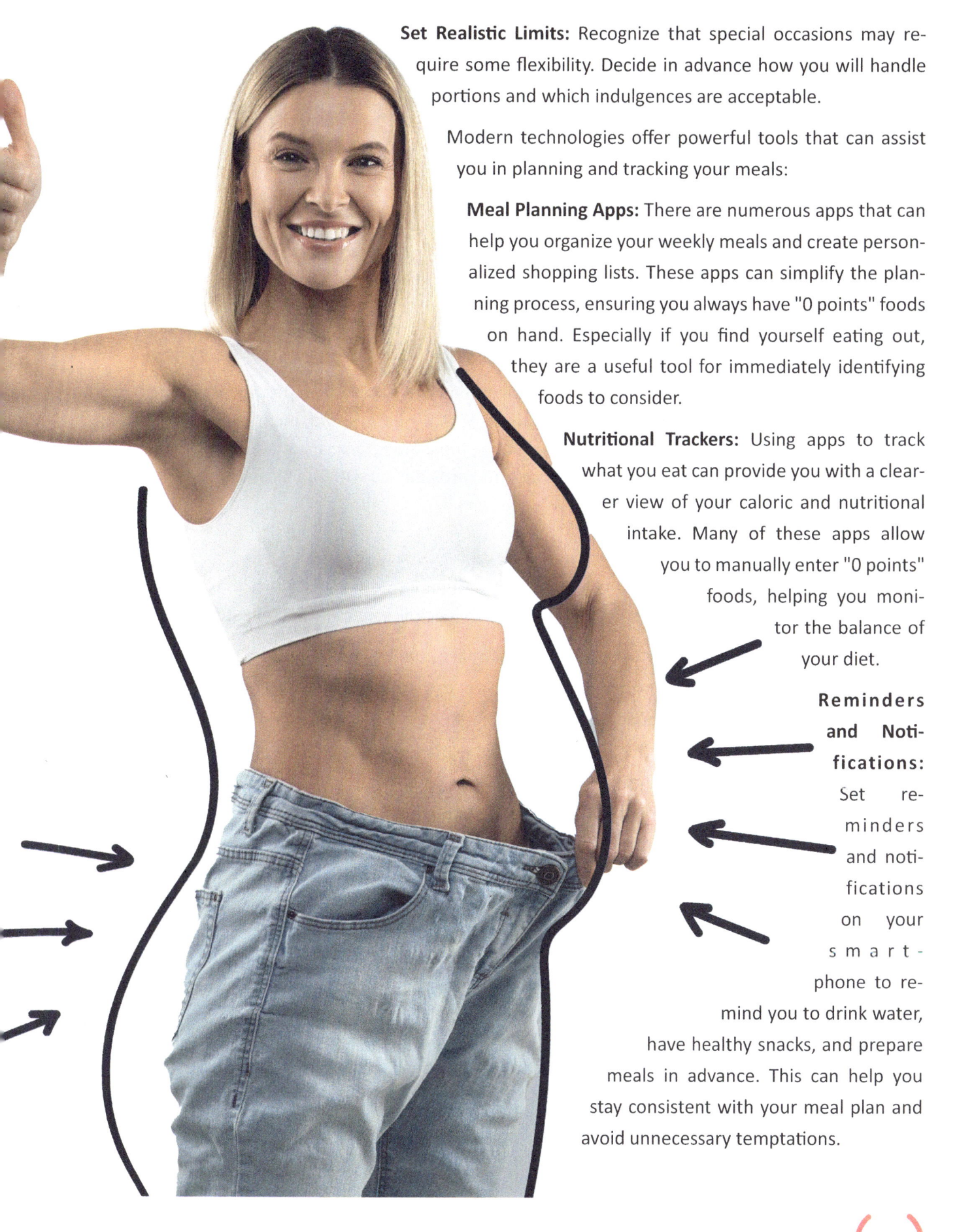

Set Realistic Limits: Recognize that special occasions may require some flexibility. Decide in advance how you will handle portions and which indulgences are acceptable.

Modern technologies offer powerful tools that can assist you in planning and tracking your meals:

Meal Planning Apps: There are numerous apps that can help you organize your weekly meals and create personalized shopping lists. These apps can simplify the planning process, ensuring you always have "0 points" foods on hand. Especially if you find yourself eating out, they are a useful tool for immediately identifying foods to consider.

Nutritional Trackers: Using apps to track what you eat can provide you with a clearer view of your caloric and nutritional intake. Many of these apps allow you to manually enter "0 points" foods, helping you monitor the balance of your diet.

Reminders and Notifications: Set reminders and notifications on your smartphone to remind you to drink water, have healthy snacks, and prepare meals in advance. This can help you stay consistent with your meal plan and avoid unnecessary temptations.

Chapter 4: Overcoming Common Challenges

Common Challenges in the "0 Points" Diet

Adopting a new diet can present a series of challenges, and the "0 points" diet is no exception. Even though it offers more freedom compared to other diets, there are still obstacles you might encounter. Among these, the most common difficulties include managing hunger, meal monotony, and maintaining long-term motivation. In this chapter, I will address these challenges and provide you with practical tools to overcome them.

Managing Hunger

One of the main challenges many people face when starting a new diet is managing hunger. Even with the abundance of "0 points" foods, you may find it difficult to feel full, especially in the first few days of transition.

- **Include Protein in Every Meal:** Protein is essential for feeling fuller for longer. Make sure each meal contains a source of lean protein such as chicken, fish, tofu, or legumes.
- **Fiber and Water:** Fiber, abundant in fruits, vegetables, and legumes, can help maintain satiety. Always pair your meals with plenty of water, which helps to swell the fiber in the digestive tract, increasing the feeling of fullness.
- **Plan Healthy Snacks:** Do not ignore hunger between meals. Plan snacks based on "0 points" foods like carrots, cucumbers, or fresh fruit. These snacks can help keep blood sugar levels stable and prevent overeating during main meals.

Variety in the Diet

Another common challenge is meal monotony. Eating the same foods every day can become boring and lead to the temptation to deviate from the meal plan.

- **Experiment with New Recipes:** One of the keys to maintaining interest in the diet is experimenting with new recipes. In the second part of the book, you will find a wide range of recipes that use "0 points" foods in creative and delicious ways.
- **Use Different Cooking Techniques:** Varying cooking techniques can completely transform the taste and texture of foods. Try grilling, baking, steaming, or sautéing to keep meals interesting.

- **Incorporate Spices and Herbs:** Spices and herbs can add flavor to your dishes without adding calories. Here are some options to consider:

Basil: Perfect for salads, tomato dishes, and as a garnish for soups.

Rosemary: Great for roasts, potatoes, and chicken dishes.

Thyme: Ideal for soups, stews, and fish dishes.

Oregano: Adds a Mediterranean touch to salads, pizzas, and grilled meats.

Parsley: Versatile and fresh, it can be used in almost any dish for a touch of freshness.

Coriander: Ideal for Asian and Mexican dishes like sauces, salads, and grilled meats.

Turmeric: An anti-inflammatory spice that can be added to curries, soups, and smoothies.

Cumin: Perfect for Mexican dishes, curries, and soups.

Paprika: Adds color and flavor to meats, soups, and stews.

Cayenne Pepper: Great for adding a bit of spiciness to your dishes.

Ginger: Used fresh or powdered, it's ideal for Asian dishes, soups, and smoothies.

Cinnamon: Perfect for sweet dishes, cooked fruit, and even savory dishes like chili.

Using a combination of these spices and herbs can transform a simple dish into a rich and varied culinary experience, keeping your interest in the diet and helping you avoid monotony.

Tips for Maintaining Motivation and Long-Term Adherence to the Diet Plan

Maintaining long-term motivation is essential for the success of your diet. Here are some strategies to stay focused and motivated:

- **Set Realistic Goals:** Define clear and achievable goals for your weight loss and overall health. Realistic goals help you stay motivated and celebrate small successes along the way.
- **Monitor Progress:** Keep track of your progress with a food diary or tracking app. Recording what you eat, how much you exercise, and how you feel can help you identify patterns and stay focused.
- **Find an Accountability Partner:** Having someone to share your journey with can make a big difference. Whether it's a friend, family member, or an online support group, an accountability partner can offer encouragement and support during difficult times.
- **Reward Yourself:** Reward your successes with something other than food. It could be a new book, a day at the spa, or a nature hike. Non-food rewards can reinforce your determination without compromising your health goals.
- **Maintain Flexibility:** Life is full of unexpected events, and there will be times when deviating from the plan is inevitable. Accept that this is part of the process and get back on track as soon as possible without guilt. The key is consistency in the long term, not perfection every single day.

Chapter 5: Integrating Physical Activity

The Importance of Exercise in Combination with the "0 Points" Diet

Integrating physical activity with the "0 points" diet not only accelerates weight loss but also improves overall health and well-being. **Exercise helps burn calories, increases metabolism, and promotes the maintenance of muscle mass, which is essential for an efficient metabolism.** Additionally, regular physical activity can improve mood, reduce stress, and increase daily energy, making it easier to adhere to the dietary plan in the long term.

To obtain the maximum benefits from physical activity in combination with the "0 points" diet, it is important to choose activities that you enjoy and that match your fitness level. Here are some options:

- **Walking:** One of the simplest and most accessible forms of exercise. **Walking daily, even just for 30 minutes, can improve cardiovascular health and help maintain weight.**
- **Resistance Training:** Weight lifting, exercises with resistance bands, or using your own body weight (like push-ups and squats) can help build and maintain muscle mass, essential for an active metabolism.
- **Yoga:** Besides improving flexibility and strength, **yoga can reduce stress and improve mental well-being**, contributing to a more balanced view of health.
- **Cycling:** Whether on the road, mountain, or stationary bike, **cycling is a great way to improve cardiovascular endurance and burn calories.**
- **Swimming:** A low-impact exercise that is gentle on the joints, **swimming can be an excellent choice for improving strength and cardiovascular endurance.**
- **High-Intensity Interval Training (HIIT):** Short, intense exercise sessions that alternate periods of high effort with recovery periods. HIIT is effective for burning fat and improving fitness in relatively short times.

Tips for Incorporating Physical Activity into Your Daily Routine, Regardless of Fitness Level

Incorporating physical activity into your daily routine can seem challenging, but with some simple adjustments, it can become a natural part of your day:

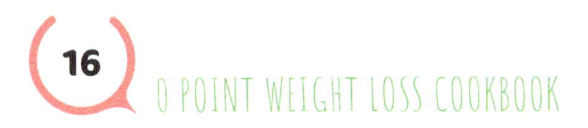

- **Start Small:** If you are new to exercise, **begin with short sessions and gradually increase the duration and intensity.** Even a 10-minute walk can make a difference if done regularly.
- **Be Consistent:** Find a time of day that works best for you and try to maintain that routine. **Whether it's early in the morning, during lunch breaks, or after work, consistency is key.**
- **Take Advantage of Every Opportunity: Incorporate movement into your day naturally.** Use stairs instead of the elevator, park further from the entrance, or take short walks during breaks.
- **Find a Workout Partner:** Having someone to exercise with can increase motivation and make physical activity more enjoyable. It can be a friend, family member, or even a workout group.
- **Set Realistic Goals:** Establish achievable goals and celebrate your progress. **This can keep you motivated and encourage you to continue.**
- **Listen to Your Body:** It is important to listen to your body and not overdo it. **If you feel pain or excessive fatigue, take the time to recover.**

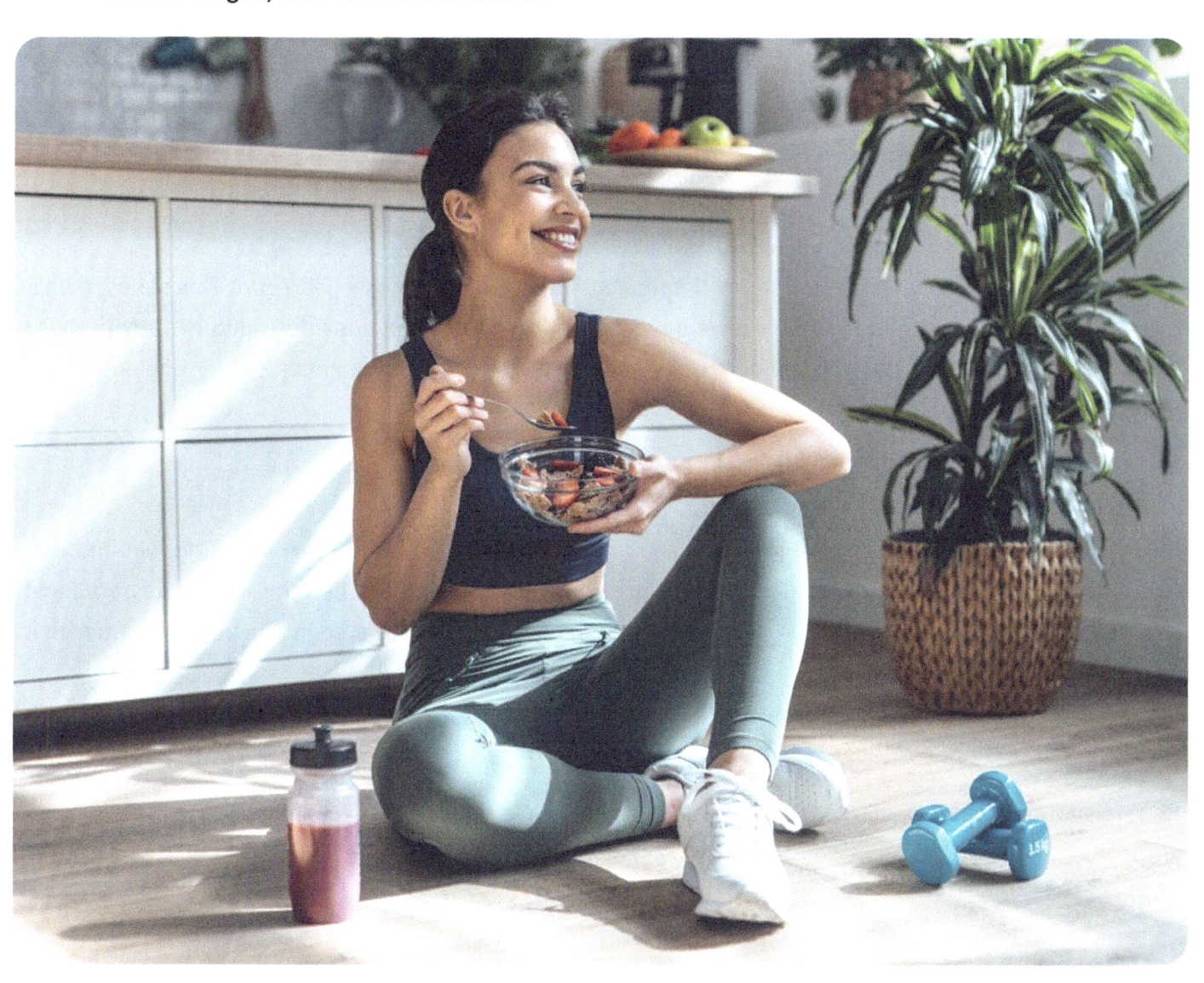

Chapter 6: Introduction to Recipes

We have taken a significant journey in understanding and implementing the "0 points" diet. We have explored the fundamental principles of this dietary approach, identified "0 points" foods, discussed meal planning and portion management, addressed common challenges, and integrated physical activity. You are now equipped with the knowledge necessary to adopt a healthy and sustainable lifestyle. **The key to success with the "0 points" diet is the simplicity and flexibility it offers, allowing you to enjoy a variety of nutritious foods without the burden of constant calorie counting.**

Preparing for Recipes

You are ready to take the next step: putting into practice everything you have learned with a series of delicious "0 points" recipes. **These recipes have been created to be not only nutritious and healthy but also simple to prepare and tasty.** They are designed to help you vary your diet, maintain satiety, and enjoy food without worrying about excess calories.

Structure of Recipes

The recipes that follow are divided into different categories to facilitate meal planning. **You will find sections dedicated to nutritious breakfasts, light lunches, substantial dinners, healthy snacks, desserts, and beverages.** Each recipe includes easily obtainable ingredients and step-by-step instructions to ensure that preparation is simple and enjoyable.

Kitchen Tips

Before starting with the recipes, here are some practical tips to optimize your culinary experience:

- **Organization:** Before you start cooking, make sure you have all the necessary ingredients and kitchen tools at hand. This makes the preparation process smoother and more enjoyable.
- **Advance Preparation:** Consider preparing some ingredients in advance, such as chopped vegetables or marinated proteins. This will help you save time during the week.

- **Exploring Flavors:** Do not be afraid to experiment with the spices and herbs we discussed. Adding unique flavors can transform a simple dish into something extraordinary.
- **Adaptability:** The provided recipes can be easily adapted to your personal tastes or the seasonal availability of ingredients. Feel free to make substitutions and additions to create dishes you love.

With the knowledge acquired and the recipes that follow, you are ready to embark on a culinary adventure that will not only help you achieve your weight loss goals but also enjoy every meal along the way. **Remember, food is an experience of pleasure as well as nutrition. Enjoy the process of exploring and discovering new flavors and combinations that will help you live a healthier and more satisfying life.**

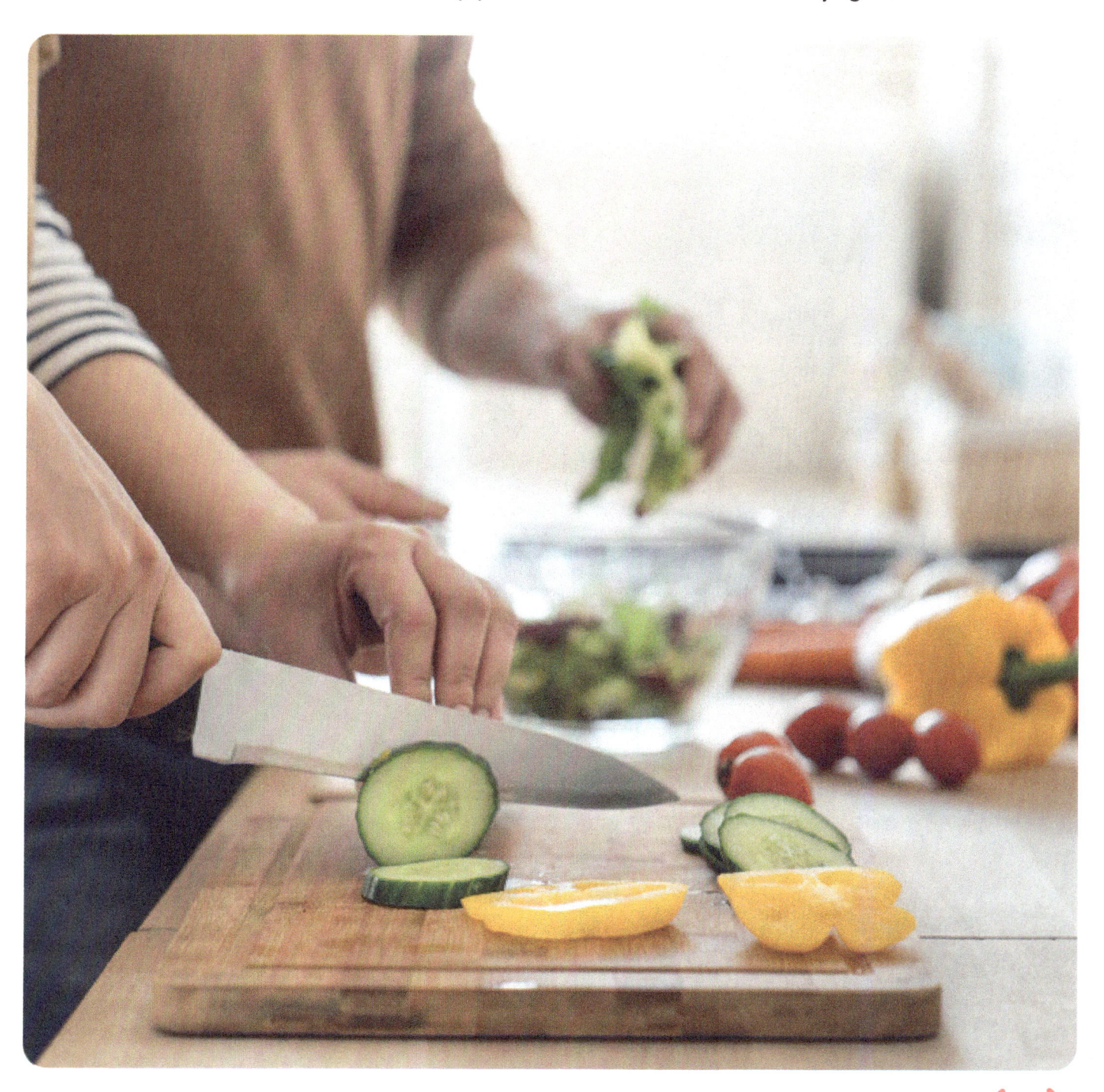

Chapter 7: Recipes

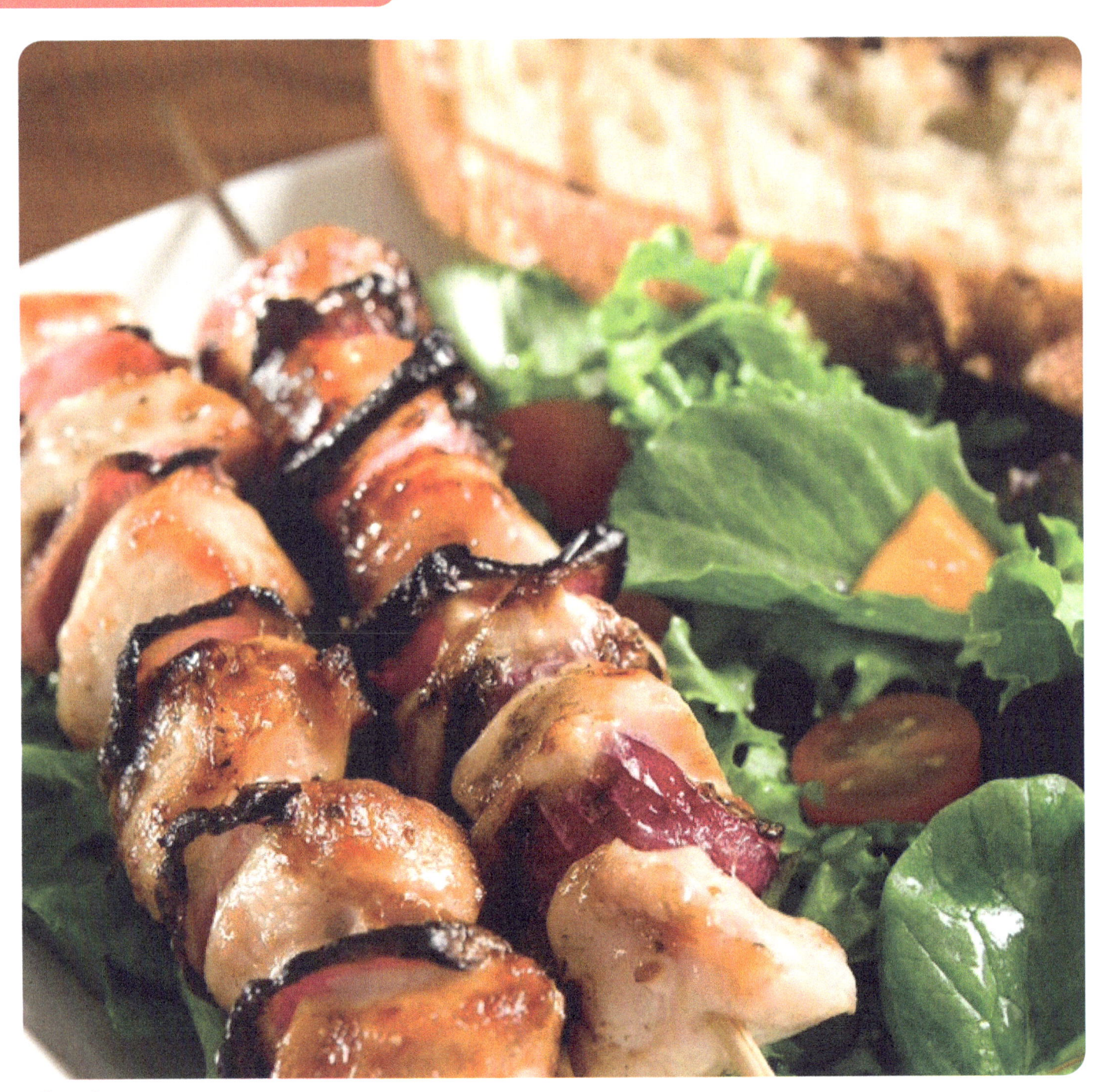

Breakfasts

Spinach and Berry Smoothie

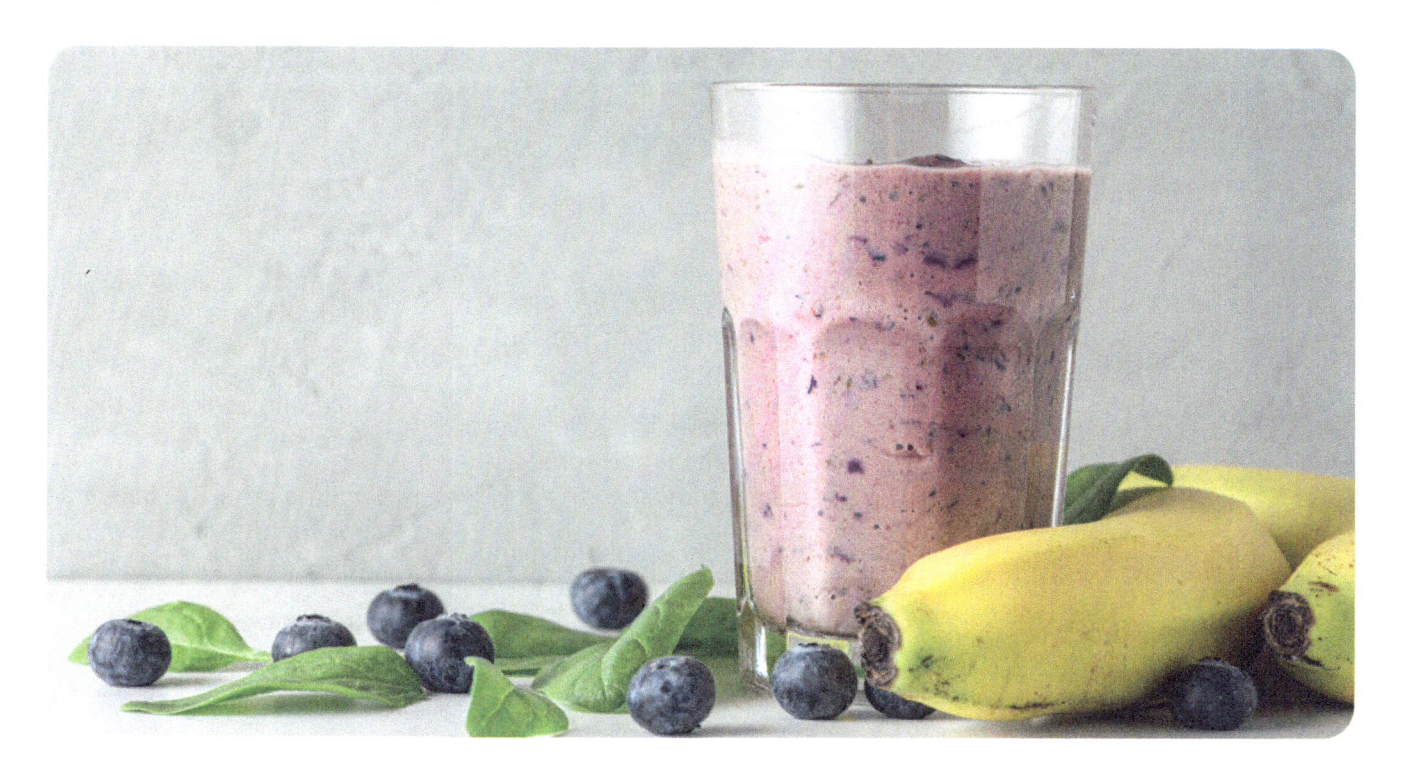

Ingredients (for 1 person):

- 1 cup fresh spinach
- 1 cup mixed berries (blueberries, strawberries, raspberries)
- 1 ripe banana
- 1 cup water or unsweetened almond milk
- 1 teaspoon chia seeds (optional)

Instructions:

1. Place the spinach, berries, banana, and water (or almond milk) in a blender.
2. Blend until smooth and consistent.
3. Add chia seeds if desired and mix well.
4. Pour into a glass and serve immediately.

NRV (per serving):

- Calories: 200
- Protein: 4g
- Fat: 2g
- Carbohydrates: 50g
- Fiber: 10g
- Sugars: 27g

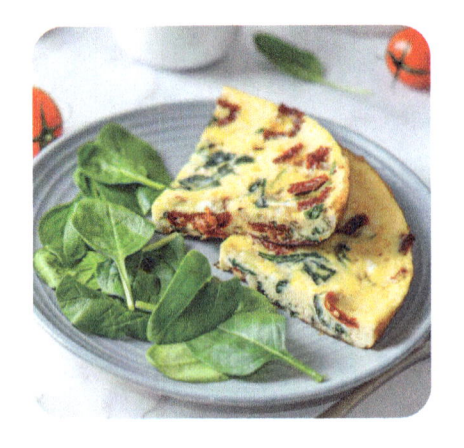

Egg White Omelette with Spinach and Tomatoes

NRV (per serving):
- Calories: 110
- Protein: 18g
- Fat: 1g
- Carbohydrates: 8g
- Fiber: 3g
- Sugars: 4g

Ingredients (for 1 person):
- 4 egg whites
- 1 cup fresh spinach
- 1 tomato, diced
- 1/4 cup chopped onion
- Salt and pepper to taste
- Non-stick cooking spray

Instructions:
1. In a bowl, whisk the egg whites with a pinch of salt and pepper.
2. Heat a non-stick skillet over medium heat and spray with cooking spray.
3. Add the chopped onion and cook until translucent.
4. Add the spinach and tomatoes and cook until the spinach is wilted.
5. Pour the egg whites into the skillet and cook until they begin to set.
6. Fold the omelette in half and cook for another 1-2 minutes.
7. Serve hot.

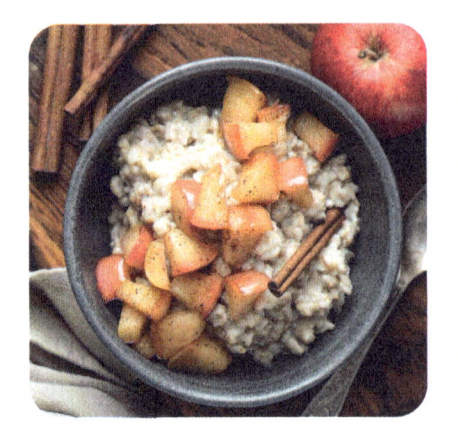

Apple Cinnamon Oatmeal

NRV (per serving):
- Calories: 180
- Protein: 5g
- Fat: 3g
- Carbohydrates: 36g
- Fiber: 6g
- Sugars: 10g

Ingredients (for 2 people):
- 1 cup rolled oats
- 2 cups water
- 1 apple, diced
- 1 teaspoon ground cinnamon
- 1 teaspoon vanilla extract (optional)

Instructions:
1. Bring the water to a boil in a pot.
2. Add the rolled oats and reduce heat to medium-low.
3. Add the diced apple, cinnamon, and vanilla extract.
4. Cook for 5-7 minutes, stirring occasionally, until the oats are tender and the porridge reaches the desired consistency.
5. Serve hot.

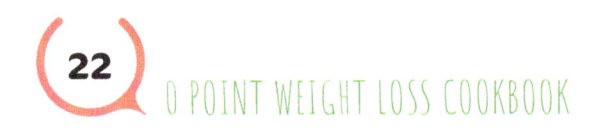

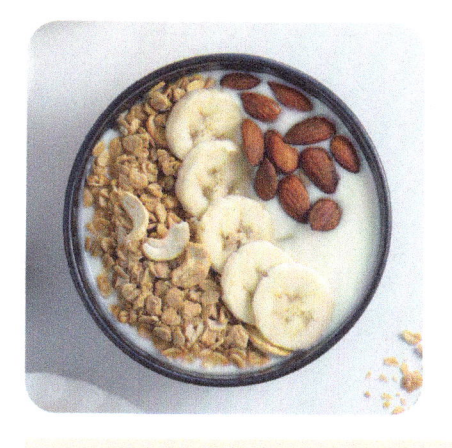

Greek Yogurt with Fruit and Nuts

NRV (per serving):
- Calories: 150
- Protein: 15g
- Fat: 3g
- Carbohydrates: 20g
- Fiber: 3g
- Sugars: 15g

Ingredients (for 1 person):
- 1 cup non-fat Greek yogurt
- 1/2 cup fresh fruit of your choice (strawberries, blueberries, kiwi)
- 1 tablespoon chopped nuts (optional)

Instructions:
1. Place the Greek yogurt in a bowl.
2. Add the fresh fruit on top of the yogurt.
3. Sprinkle the chopped nuts if desired.
4. Mix well and serve immediately.

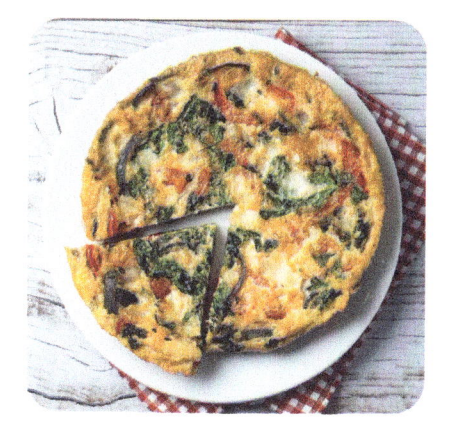

Vegetable Frittata

NRV (per serving):
- Calories: 140
- Protein: 10g
- Fat: 9g
- Carbohydrates: 6g
- Fiber: 2g
- Sugars: 3g

Ingredients (for 2 people):
- 3 whole eggs
- 1/2 cup sliced mushrooms
- 1/2 red bell pepper, diced
- 1 zucchini, sliced
- Salt and pepper to taste
- Non-stick cooking spray

Instructions:
1. In a bowl, whisk the eggs with a pinch of salt and pepper.
2. Heat a non-stick skillet over medium heat and spray with cooking spray.
3. Add the mushrooms, bell pepper, and zucchini and cook until the vegetables are tender.
4. Pour the beaten eggs into the skillet and cook until they begin to set.
5. Fold the frittata in half and cook for another 1-2 minutes.
6. Serve hot.

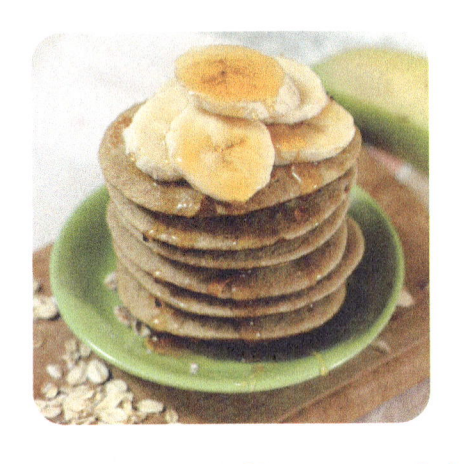

Banana Oat Pancakes

NRV (per serving):
- Calories: 220
- Protein: 8g
- Fat: 6g
- Carbohydrates: 36g
- Fiber: 5g
- Sugars: 10g

Ingredients (for 2 people):
- 1 cup oats
- 1 ripe banana
- 2 eggs
- 1/2 teaspoon vanilla extract
- 1/2 teaspoon ground cinnamon
- 1/2 teaspoon baking powder
- Non-stick cooking spray

Instructions:
1. Place the oats in a blender and blend until fine.
2. Add the banana, eggs, vanilla extract, cinnamon, and baking powder. Blend until smooth.
3. Heat a non-stick skillet over medium heat and spray with cooking spray.
4. Pour about 1/4 cup of batter for each pancake into the skillet.
5. Cook the pancakes for 2-3 minutes on each side until golden brown.
6. Serve hot, optionally with fresh fruit or Greek yogurt.

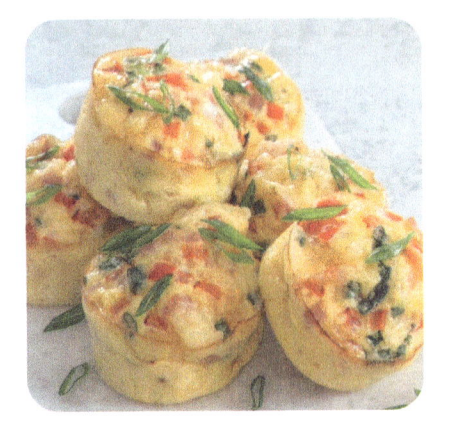

Egg and Vegetable Muffins

NRV (per serving, 2 muffins):
- Calories: 140
- Protein: 12g
- Fat: 8g
- Carbohydrates: 6g
- Fiber: 2g
- Sugars: 3g

Greek Yogurt

Ingr. (for 6 muffins, 3 servings):
- 6 eggs
- 1/2 cup chopped fresh spinach
- 1/4 cup chopped sun-dried tomatoes
- 1/4 cup chopped onion
- 1/4 cup chopped red bell pepper
- Salt and pepper to taste
- Non-stick cooking spray

Instructions:
1. Preheat the oven to 350°F (175°C) and spray a muffin tin with cooking spray.
2. In a large bowl, whisk the eggs with a pinch of salt and pepper.
3. Add the spinach, sun-dried tomatoes, onion, and red bell pepper to the eggs and mix well.
4. Pour the egg mixture into the muffin tins, filling them about 3/4 full.
5. Bake for 20-25 minutes or until the egg muffins are puffed and golden brown.
6. Let cool slightly before serving.

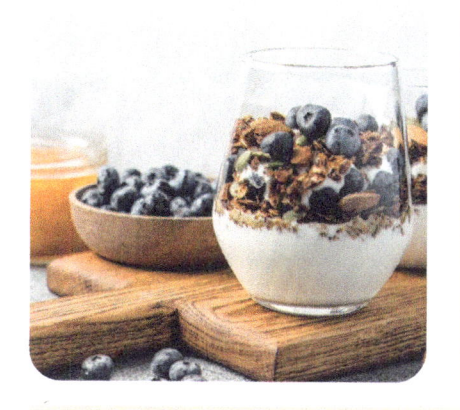

and Muesli Parfait

NRV (per serving):
- Calories: 300
- Protein: 20g
- Fat: 5g
- Carbohydrates: 50g
- Fiber: 8g
- Sugars: 25g

Ingredients (for 1 person):
- 1 cup non-fat Greek yogurt
- 1/2 cup unsweetened muesli
- 1/2 cup fresh fruit (strawberries, blueberries, raspberries)
- 1 teaspoon honey (optional)

Instructions:
1. In a bowl or glass, layer the Greek yogurt.
2. Add a layer of muesli and then a layer of fresh fruit.
3. Repeat the layers until all ingredients are used up.
4. Drizzle honey on top if desired.
5. Serve immediately.

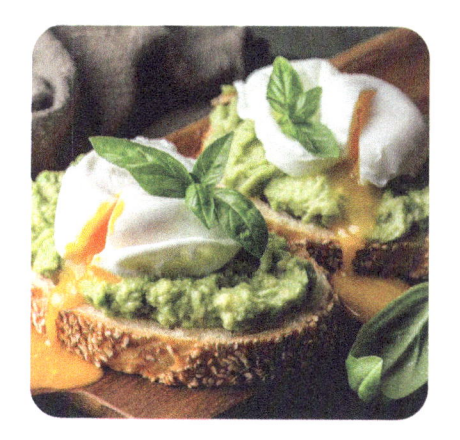

Avocado Toast with Poached Eggs

NRV (per serving):
- Calories: 290
- Protein: 10g
- Fat: 22g
- Carbohydrates: 20g
- Fiber: 8g
- Sugars: 2g

Ingredients (for 2 people):
- 2 slices whole-grain bread
- 1 ripe avocado
- 2 eggs
- 1 tablespoon white vinegar
- Salt and pepper to taste
- Red pepper flakes (optional)

Instructions:
1. Toast the slices of bread until golden brown.
2. Peel and mash the avocado, then spread it on the toasted bread. Add salt and pepper to taste.
3. Bring a pot of water to a boil and add the white vinegar.
4. Reduce the heat to medium and create a whirlpool in the water with a spoon.
5. Crack an egg into a small bowl and gently slide the egg into the whirlpool. Cook for 3-4 minutes, then remove the egg with a slotted spoon.
6. Repeat with the other egg.
7. Place a poached egg on each slice of bread with avocado.
8. Add red pepper flakes if desired and serve immediately.

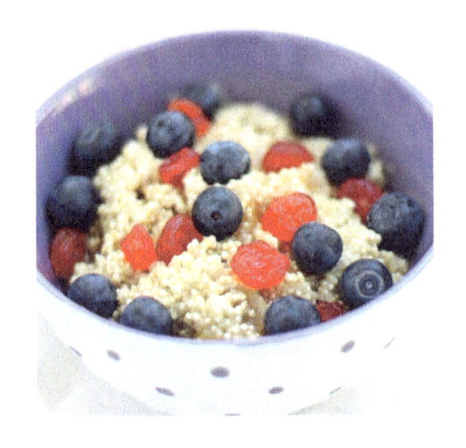

Quinoa Porridge with Berries

NRV (per serving):
- Calories: 250
- Protein: 7g
- Fat: 4g
- Carbohydrates: 50g
- Fiber: 7g
- Sugars: 10g

Ingredients (for 2 people):
- 1 cup quinoa
- 2 cups water
- 1 cup mixed berries (blueberries, strawberries, raspberries)
- 1 teaspoon ground cinnamon
- 1 tablespoon honey (optional)

Instructions:
1. Rinse the quinoa under cold running water.
2. Bring the water to a boil in a pot and add the quinoa.
3. Reduce the heat to medium-low, cover, and cook for 15 minutes or until the quinoa is tender and the water is absorbed.
4. Add the cinnamon and mix well.
5. Divide the cooked quinoa into bowls and add the berries.
6. Drizzle honey on top if desired and serve warm.

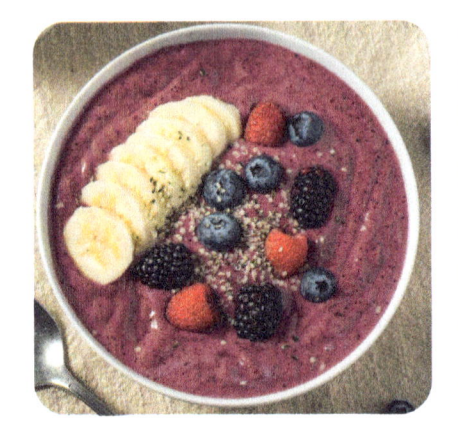

Berry Smoothie Bowl

NRV (per serving):
- Calories: 280
- Protein: 5g
- Fat: 7g
- Carbohydrates: 56g
- Fiber: 12g
- Sugars: 28g

Ingredients (for 1 person):
- 1 cup frozen mixed berries (blueberries, strawberries, raspberries)
- 1 ripe banana
- 1/2 cup unsweetened almond milk
- 1 tablespoon chia seeds
- 1/4 cup unsweetened granola (optional)
- 1 tablespoon shredded coconut (optional)

Instructions:
1. Place the berries, banana, and almond milk in a blender.
2. Blend until smooth and thick.
3. Pour the mixture into a bowl.
4. Add chia seeds, granola, and shredded coconut as toppings if desired.
5. Serve immediately.

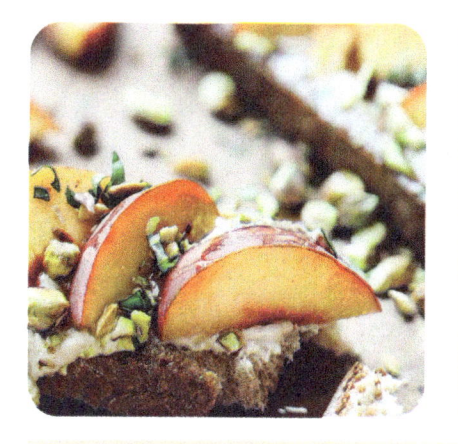

Whole Wheat Toast with Ricotta and Fruit

NRV (per serving):
- Calories: 220
- Protein: 11g
- Fat: 4g
- Carbohydrates: 34g
- Fiber: 6g
- Sugars: 15g

Ingredients (for 2 people):
- 2 slices whole-grain bread
- 1/2 cup fat-free ricotta
- 1 peach, sliced
- 1 tablespoon honey
- 1 teaspoon chia seeds (optional)

Instructions:
1. Toast the slices of bread until golden brown.
2. Spread the ricotta on the toasted bread.
3. Arrange the peach slices on top of the ricotta.
4. Drizzle honey on top and add chia seeds if desired.
5. Serve immediately.

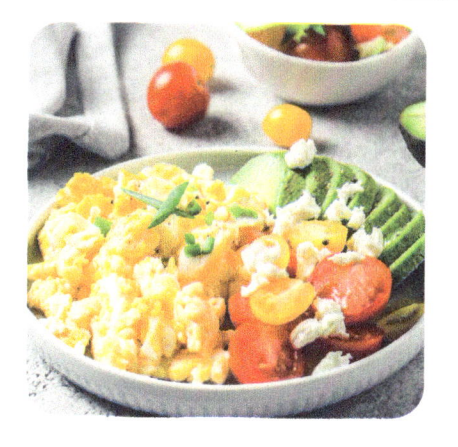

Scrambled Eggs with Avocado and Tomato

NRV (per serving):
- Calories: 250
- Protein: 12g
- Fat: 18g
- Carbohydrates: 12g
- Fiber: 6g
- Sugars: 3g

Ingredients (for 2 people):
- 4 eggs
- 1 ripe avocado, sliced
- 1 tomato, diced
- 1/4 cup chopped red onion
- Salt and pepper to taste
- Non-stick cooking spray

Instructions:
1. In a bowl, whisk the eggs with a pinch of salt and pepper.
2. Heat a non-stick skillet over medium heat and spray with cooking spray.
3. Add the red onion and cook until translucent.
4. Pour the beaten eggs into the skillet and cook, stirring continuously, until scrambled and cooked through.
5. Place the scrambled eggs on a plate and top with the sliced avocado and diced tomato.
6. Serve immediately.

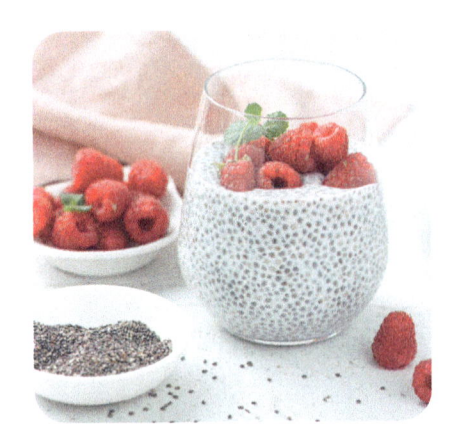

Chia Pudding with Almond Milk and Fruit

NRV (per serving):
- Calories: 200
- Protein: 5g
- Fat: 10g
- Carbohydrates: 25g
- Fiber: 12g
- Sugars: 10g

Ingredients (for 2 people):
- 1/4 cup chia seeds
- 1 cup unsweetened almond milk
- 1 teaspoon vanilla extract
- 1 tablespoon honey (optional)
- 1/2 cup fresh fruit (blueberries, strawberries, kiwi)

Instructions:
1. In a bowl, mix the chia seeds, almond milk, and vanilla extract.
2. Add honey if desired and mix well.
3. Cover the bowl and refrigerate for at least 4 hours or overnight.
4. When ready to serve, divide the chia pudding into two bowls and top with fresh fruit.
5. Serve immediately.

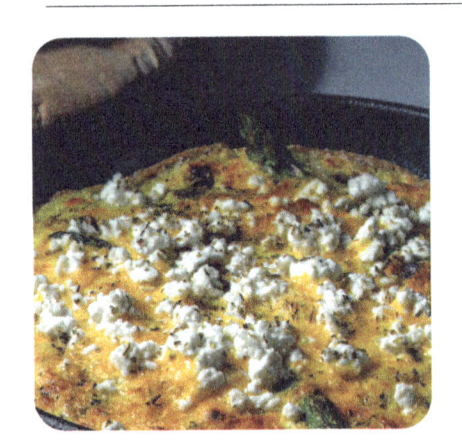

Asparagus and Feta Frittata

NRV (per serving):
- Calories: 210
- Protein: 14g
- Fat: 14g
- Carbohydrates: 5g
- Fiber: 2g
- Sugars: 2g

Ingredients (for 2 people):
- 4 eggs
- 1/2 cup chopped asparagus
- 1/4 cup crumbled feta
- 1/4 cup chopped green onion
- Salt and pepper to taste
- Non-stick cooking spray

Instructions:
1. In a bowl, whisk the eggs with a pinch of salt and pepper.
2. Heat a non-stick skillet over medium heat and spray with cooking spray.
3. Add the asparagus and cook until tender.
4. Pour the beaten eggs into the skillet and cook until they begin to set.
5. Add the crumbled feta and green onion on top of the eggs.
6. Fold the frittata in half and cook for another 1-2 minutes.
7. Serve hot.

Lunches

Grilled Chicken Salad

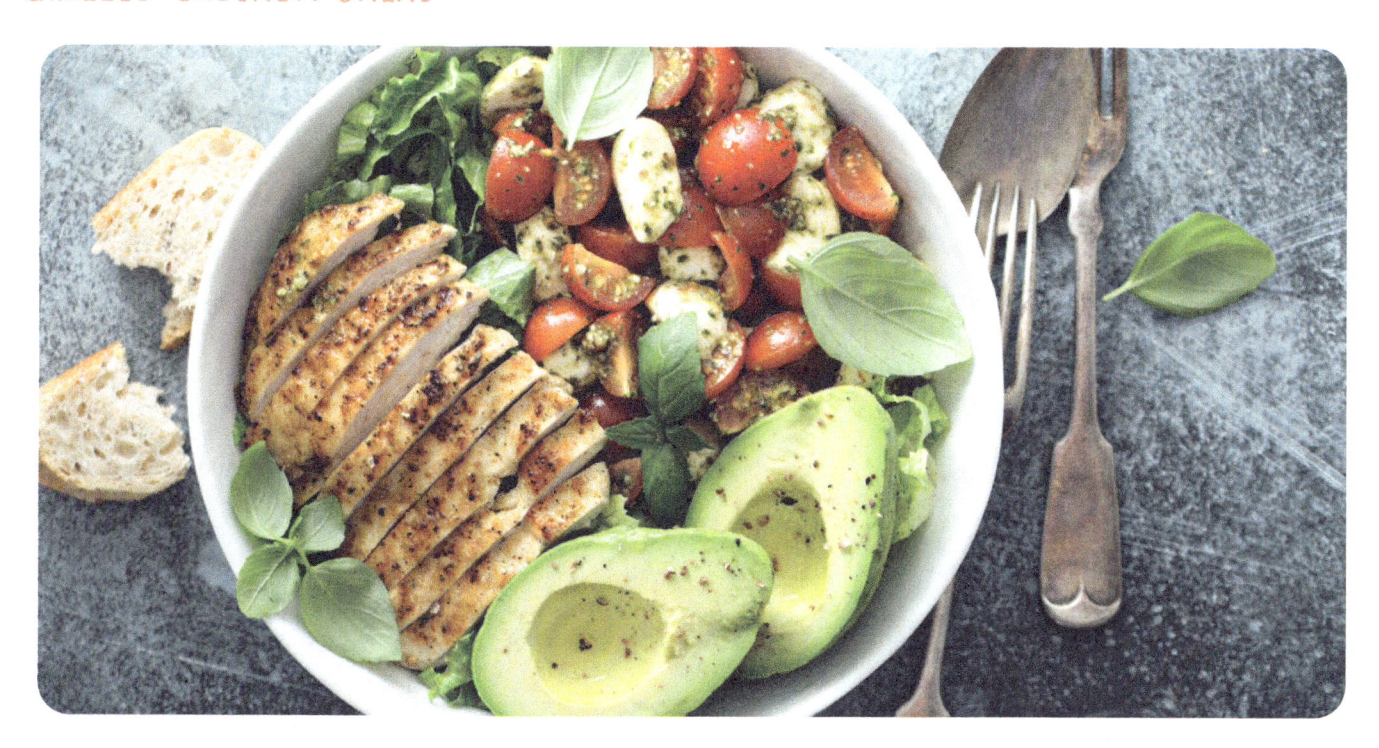

Ingredients (for 2 people):
- 2 skinless chicken breasts
- 4 cups mixed lettuce
- 1 cup cherry tomatoes, halved
- 1 avocado, diced
- 1/4 cup red onion, thinly sliced
- 1/4 cup cucumber, sliced
- 2 tablespoons olive oil
- Juice of 1 lemon
- Salt and pepper to taste

Instructions:
1. Preheat a grill to medium-high heat. Season the chicken breasts with salt and pepper.
2. Grill the chicken for 6-7 minutes per side or until fully cooked. Let rest for 5 minutes, then slice.
3. In a large bowl, combine the lettuce, cherry tomatoes, avocado, red onion, and cucumber.
4. Add the grilled chicken on top of the salad.
5. In a small bowl, whisk together the olive oil, lemon juice, salt, and pepper.
6. Pour the dressing over the salad and mix well.
7. Serve immediately.

NRV (per serving):
- Calories: 350
- Protein: 30g
- Fat: 22g
- Carbohydrates: 12g
- Fiber: 7g
- Sugars: 4g

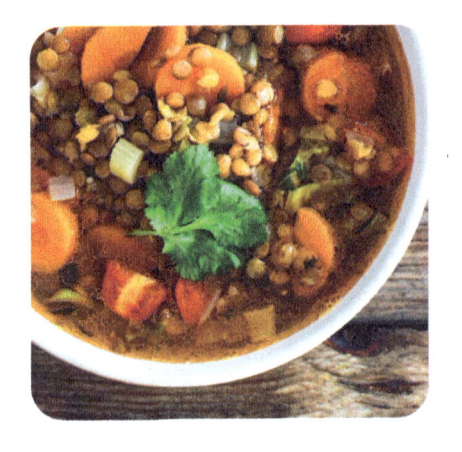

Lentil and Vegetable Soup

NRV (per serving):
- Calories: 250
- Protein: 12g
- Fat: 4g
- Carbohydrates: 40g
- Fiber: 16g
- Sugars: 8g

Ingredients (for 4 people):
- 1 cup dry green lentils
- 1 onion, chopped
- 2 carrots, sliced
- 2 celery stalks, sliced
- 2 cloves garlic, minced
- 1 zucchini, diced
- 1 large tomato, diced
- 6 cups low-sodium vegetable broth
- 1 teaspoon ground cumin
- 1 teaspoon paprika
- 1 tablespoon olive oil
- Salt and pepper to taste
- Fresh parsley, chopped (optional)

Instructions:
1. In a large pot, heat the olive oil over medium heat. Add the onion, carrots, celery, and garlic. Cook until the vegetables are tender, about 5 minutes.
2. Add the lentils, zucchini, tomato, vegetable broth, cumin, and paprika. Bring to a boil.
3. Reduce heat, cover, and simmer for 30-35 minutes or until the lentils are tender.
4. Season with salt and pepper to taste.
5. Serve hot, garnished with fresh parsley if desired.

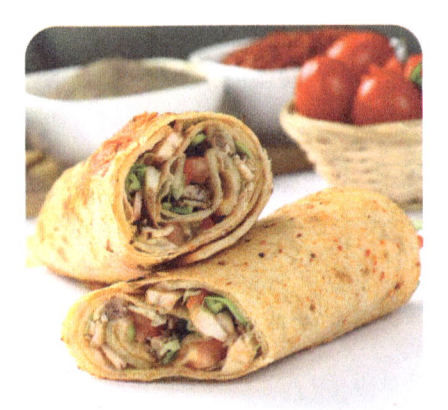

Turkey and Vegetable Wrap

NRV (per serving):
- Calories: 350
- Protein: 20g
- Fat: 15g
- Carbohydrates: 35g
- Fiber: 10g
- Sugars: 4g

Ingredients (for 2 people):
- 4 whole-wheat tortillas
- 8 slices of roasted turkey breast (about 8 oz)
- 1 cup chopped romaine lettuce
- 1/2 cup shredded carrots
- 1/2 cup sliced red bell pepper
- 1/4 cup hummus
- 1 avocado, sliced
- Juice of 1/2 lemon
- Salt and pepper to taste

Instructions:
1. Spread a thin layer of hummus on each tortilla.
2. Add 2 slices of turkey to each tortilla.
3. Evenly distribute the lettuce, carrots, bell pepper, and avocado on each tortilla.
4. Drizzle with lemon juice and season with salt and pepper to taste.
5. Roll the tortillas tightly, cut in half, and serve.

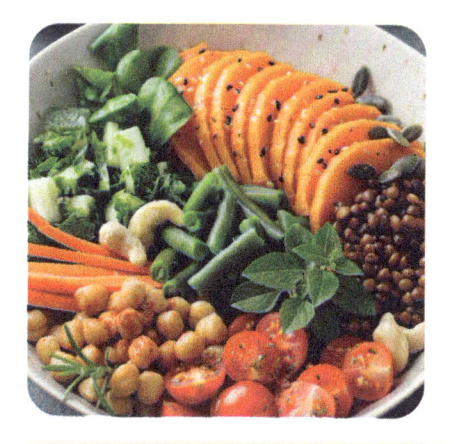

Quinoa Salad with Chickpeas and Vegetables

NRV (per serving):
- Calories: 300
- Protein: 10g
- Fat: 12g
- Carbohydrates: 40g
- Fiber: 8g
- Sugars: 4g

Ingredients (for 4 people):
- 1 cup quinoa
- 2 cups water
- 1 cup cooked chickpeas
- 1 cup sliced cucumber
- 1 cup cherry tomatoes, halved
- 1/4 cup red onion, chopped
- 1/4 cup black olives, sliced
- 2 tablespoons olive oil
- Juice of 1 lemon
- Salt and pepper to taste
- Fresh mint leaves, chopped (optional)

Instructions:
1. Rinse the quinoa under cold running water.
2. In a pot, bring the water to a boil and add the quinoa. Reduce heat to medium-low, cover, and cook for 15 minutes or until the quinoa is tender and the water is absorbed. Let cool.
3. In a large bowl, combine the cooked quinoa, chickpeas, cucumber, cherry tomatoes, red onion, and black olives.
4. In a small bowl, whisk together the olive oil, lemon juice, salt, and pepper.
5. Pour the dressing over the salad and mix well.
6. Add fresh mint leaves if desired and serve.

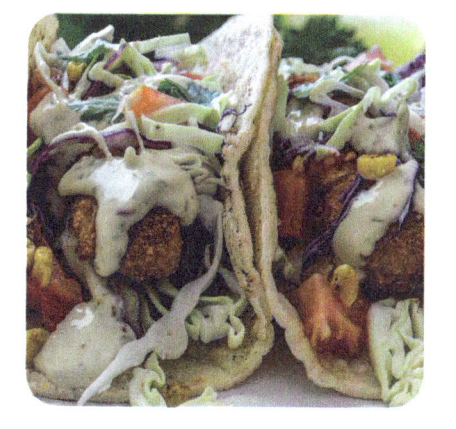

Fish Tacos with Avocado Sauce

NRV (per serving):
- Calories: 300
- Protein: 22g
- Fat: 12g
- Carbohydrates: 30g
- Fiber: 8g
- Sugars: 4g

Ingredients (for 4 people):
- 1 lb white fish fillets (tilapia, cod, etc.)
- 8 corn tortillas
- 1 avocado, mashed
- 1/2 cup non-fat Greek yogurt
- Juice of 1 lime
- 1/4 cup fresh cilantro, chopped
- 2 cups shredded red cabbage
- 1/2 cup shredded carrots
- 1 teaspoon ground cumin
- 1 teaspoon paprika
- Salt and pepper to taste
- Non-stick cooking spray

Instructions:
1. Season the fish fillets with cumin, paprika, salt, and pepper.
2. Heat a non-stick skillet over medium heat and spray with cooking spray.
3. Cook the fish fillets for 3-4 minutes per side or until cooked through and flaky. Let cool slightly and then break into pieces.
4. In a small bowl, mix the mashed avocado, Greek yogurt, lime juice, and cilantro. Season with salt and pepper.
5. Warm the corn tortillas in a skillet or microwave.
6. Divide the fish among the tortillas, and top with shredded cabbage, carrots, and avocado sauce.
7. Serve immediately.

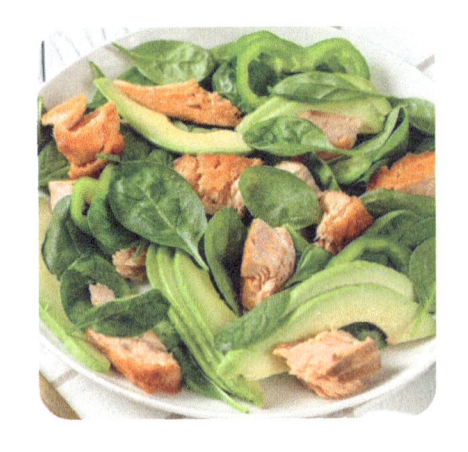

Spinach Salad with Salmon and Avocado

NRV (per serving):
- Calories: 450
- Protein: 30g
- Fat: 30g
- Carbohydrates: 12g
- Fiber: 8g
- Sugars: 2g

Ingredients (for 2 people):
- 2 salmon fillets (about 6 oz each)
- 4 cups fresh spinach
- 1 avocado, diced
- 1/2 cup cherry tomatoes, halved
- 1/4 cup red onion, thinly sliced
- 1 tablespoon olive oil
- Juice of 1/2 lemon
- Salt and pepper to taste

Instructions:
1. Preheat a non-stick skillet over medium-high heat. Season the salmon fillets with salt and pepper.
2. Cook the salmon for 4-5 minutes per side or until cooked to your preference. Let cool slightly and then break into pieces.
3. In a large bowl, combine the spinach, avocado, cherry tomatoes, and red onion.
4. Add the salmon pieces on top of the salad.
5. In a small bowl, whisk together the olive oil, lemon juice, salt, and pepper.
6. Pour the dressing over the salad and mix gently.
7. Serve immediately.

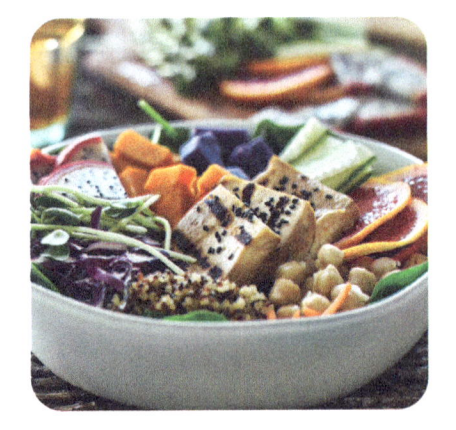

Buddha Bowl with Tofu and Vegetable

NRV (per serving):
- Calories: 480
- Protein: 20g
- Fat: 24g
- Carbohydrates: 48g
- Fiber: 12g
- Sugars: 4g

Ingredients (for 2 people):
- 1 cup quinoa
- 2 cups water
- 1 block tofu (about 14 oz), cubed
- 1 cup broccoli florets
- 1 carrot, thinly sliced
- 1 red bell pepper, sliced
- 1 avocado, sliced
- 2 tablespoons low-sodium soy sauce
- 1 tablespoon sesame oil
- 1 teaspoon fresh ginger, grated
- 1 tablespoon sesame seeds

Instructions:
1. Rinse the quinoa under cold running water.
2. In a pot, bring the water to a boil and add the quinoa. Reduce heat to medium-low, cover, and cook for 15 minutes or until the quinoa is tender and the water is absorbed. Let cool.
3. Heat the sesame oil in a non-stick skillet over medium-high heat. Add the tofu and cook until golden and crispy on all sides, about 10 minutes.
4. Add the grated ginger and soy sauce to the tofu, stirring well to coat evenly. Cook for another 2 minutes.
5. Divide the cooked quinoa into two bowls. Add the broccoli, carrot, red bell pepper, and avocado.
6. Top with the tofu.
7. Sprinkle with sesame seeds and serve.

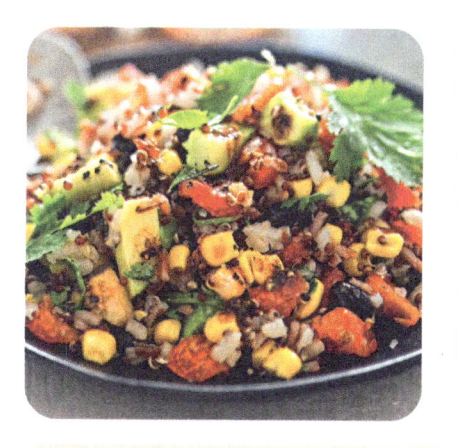

Black Bean and Corn Salad

NRV (per serving):
- Calories: 250
- Protein: 8g
- Fat: 12g
- Carbohydrates: 32g
- Fiber: 10g
- Sugars: 4g

Ingredients (for 4 people):
- 1 can black beans (15 oz), drained and rinsed
- 1 can corn (15 oz), drained
- 1 red bell pepper, diced
- 1 green bell pepper, diced
- 1/2 cup red onion, chopped
- 1 avocado, diced
- Juice of 2 limes
- 2 tablespoons olive oil
- 1/4 cup fresh cilantro, chopped
- Salt and pepper to taste

Instructions:
1. In a large bowl, combine the black beans, corn, red bell pepper, green bell pepper, red onion, and avocado.
2. In a small bowl, whisk together the lime juice, olive oil, cilantro, salt, and pepper.
3. Pour the dressing over the salad and mix gently to combine.
4. Let sit for at least 10 minutes before serving to allow the flavors to meld.
5. Serve as a side dish or main course.

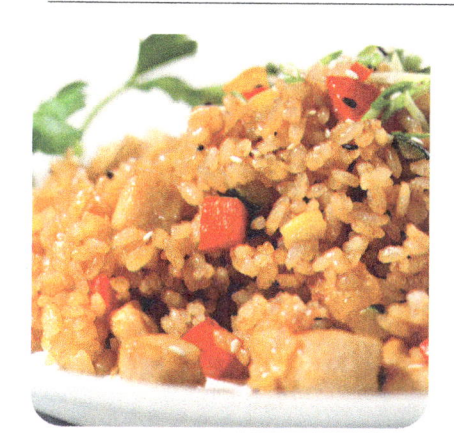

Brown Rice with Curry Vegetables

NRV (per serving):
- Calories: 350
- Protein: 8g
- Fat: 14g
- Carbohydrates: 50g
- Fiber: 6g
- Sugars: 4g

Ingredients (for 4 people):
- 1 cup brown rice
- 2 cups water
- 1 tablespoon coconut oil
- 1 onion, chopped
- 2 cloves garlic, minced
- 1 tablespoon curry powder
- 1 cup frozen peas
- 1 cup sliced carrots
- 1 cup diced zucchini
- 1 can coconut milk (13.5 oz)
- Salt and pepper to taste
- 1/4 cup fresh cilantro, chopped (optional)

Instructions:
1. Rinse the rice under cold running water.
2. In a pot, bring the water to a boil and add the brown rice. Reduce heat to medium-low, cover, and cook for 40-45 minutes or until the rice is tender and the water is absorbed. Let sit, covered, for 5 minutes.
3. In a large skillet, heat the coconut oil over medium heat. Add the onion and garlic and cook until tender, about 5 minutes.
4. Add the curry powder and cook for 1 minute, stirring constantly.
5. Add the peas, carrots, and zucchini to the skillet and cook for 5-7 minutes or until the vegetables are tender.
6. Pour in the coconut milk and bring to a simmer. Reduce heat and cook for another 5 minutes.
7. Season with salt and pepper to taste.
8. Divide the brown rice into plates and spoon the curry vegetables over the top.
9. Garnish with fresh cilantro if desired and serve.

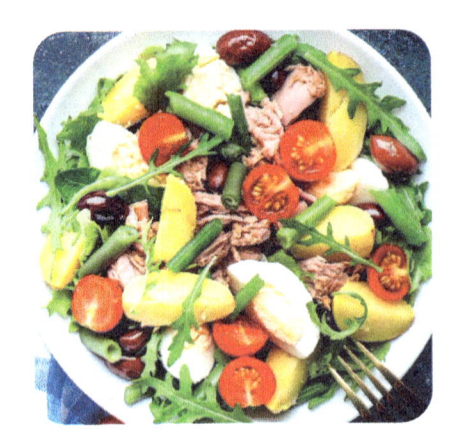

Tuna Salad with Green Beans and Potatoes

NRV (per serving):
- Calories: 300
- Protein: 18g
- Fat: 14g
- Carbohydrates: 28g
- Fiber: 6g
- Sugars: 4g

Ingredients (for 4 people):
- 1 lb new potatoes, halved
- 1/2 lb green beans, trimmed
- 2 cans tuna in water (5 oz each), drained
- 1/2 cup cherry tomatoes, halved
- 1/4 cup red onion, thinly sliced
- 1/4 cup black olives, sliced
- 2 tablespoons capers, drained
- 1/4 cup olive oil
- Juice of 1 lemon
- Salt and pepper to taste

Instructions:
1. Bring a large pot of salted water to a boil. Add the potatoes and cook for 10 minutes.
2. Add the green beans to the potatoes and cook for another 5 minutes or until the potatoes and green beans are tender. Drain and let cool.
3. In a large bowl, combine the tuna, cherry tomatoes, red onion, black olives, and capers.
4. Add the cooled potatoes and green beans to the bowl.
5. In a small bowl, whisk together the olive oil, lemon juice, salt, and pepper.
6. Pour the dressing over the salad and mix gently to combine.
7. Serve immediately or refrigerate until ready to serve.

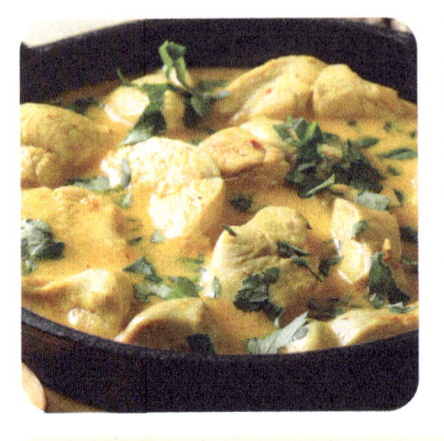

Coconut Curry Chicken

NRV (per serving):
- Calories: 350
- Protein: 22g
- Fat: 22g
- Carbohydrates: 15g
- Fiber: 4g
- Sugars: 4g

Ingredients (for 4 people):
- 1 lb chicken breast, cubed
- 1 can coconut milk (13.5 oz)
- 1 onion, chopped
- 2 cloves garlic, minced
- 1 tablespoon coconut oil
- 2 tablespoons red curry paste
- 1 red bell pepper, sliced
- 1 zucchini, diced
- 1 cup fresh spinach
- Juice of 1 lime
- Salt and pepper to taste
- Fresh cilantro, chopped (optional)

Instructions:
1. Heat the coconut oil in a large skillet over medium heat. Add the onion and garlic and cook until tender, about 5 minutes.
2. Add the curry paste and cook for 1 minute, stirring constantly.
3. Add the chicken and cook until golden on all sides, about 5-7 minutes.
4. Pour in the coconut milk and bring to a simmer.
5. Add the bell pepper and zucchini and cook for another 5 minutes or until the vegetables are tender.
6. Stir in the spinach until wilted.
7. Season with lime juice, salt, and pepper to taste.
8. Garnish with fresh cilantro if desired and serve hot.

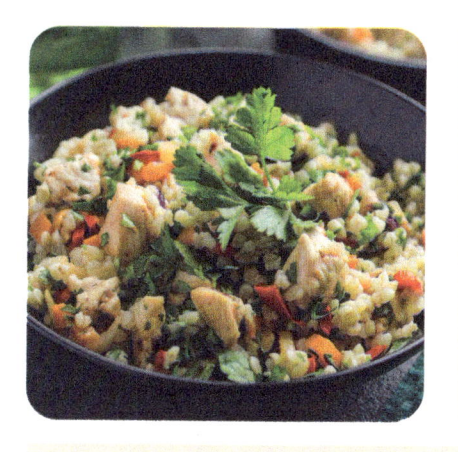

Barley Salad with Roasted Vegetables

NRV (per serving):
- Calories: 300
- Protein: 8g
- Fat: 12g
- Carbohydrates: 40g
- Fiber: 8g
- Sugars: 6g

Ingredients (for 4 people):
- 1 cup barley
- 2 cups water
- 1 red bell pepper, diced
- 1 yellow bell pepper, diced
- 1 zucchini, diced
- 1 red onion, quartered
- 2 tablespoons olive oil
- 1 tablespoon balsamic vinegar
- 1/4 cup crumbled feta cheese
- Salt and pepper to taste
- Fresh parsley, chopped (optional)

Instructions:
1. Preheat the oven to 400°F (200°C).
2. In a pot, bring the water to a boil and add the barley. Reduce heat and cook for 20-25 minutes or until the barley is tender. Drain and let cool.
3. On a baking sheet, toss the red bell pepper, yellow bell pepper, zucchini, and red onion with 1 tablespoon olive oil, salt, and pepper.
4. Roast the vegetables in the oven for 20-25 minutes or until tender and lightly caramelized.
5. In a large bowl, combine the cooked barley, roasted vegetables, feta cheese, remaining olive oil, and balsamic vinegar.
6. Season with salt and pepper to taste.
7. Add fresh parsley if desired and serve.

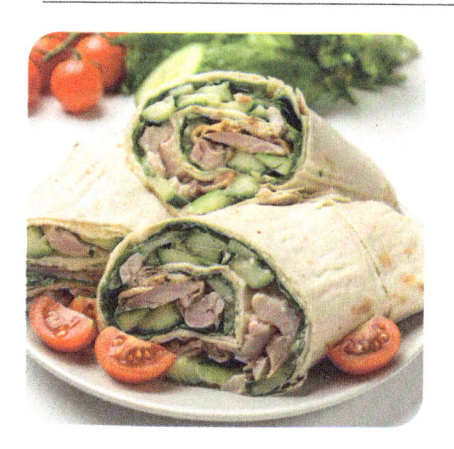

Turkey and Avocado Wrap

NRV (per serving):
- Calories: 350
- Protein: 20g
- Fat: 18g
- Carbohydrates: 30g
- Fiber: 8g
- Sugars: 4g

Ingredients (for 2 people):
- 4 whole-wheat tortillas
- 8 slices of roasted turkey breast (about 8 oz)
- 1 avocado, sliced
- 1/2 cup chopped romaine lettuce
- 1/2 cup sliced tomatoes
- 2 tablespoons light mayonnaise (optional)
- Juice of 1/2 lemon
- Salt and pepper to taste

Instructions:
1. Spread a thin layer of mayonnaise on each tortilla if using.
2. Add 2 slices of turkey to each tortilla.
3. Evenly distribute the sliced avocado, lettuce, and tomatoes on each tortilla.
4. Drizzle with lemon juice and season with salt and pepper to taste.
5. Roll the tortillas tightly, cut in half, and serve.

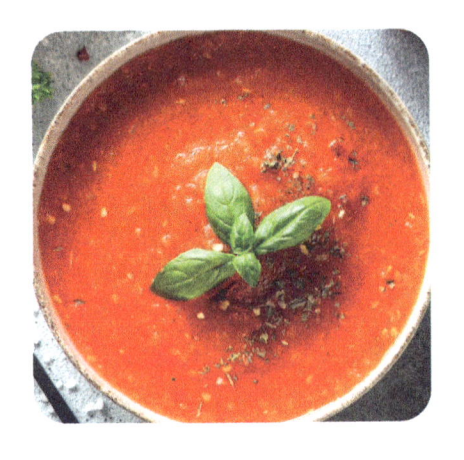

Tomato Basil Soup

NRV (per serving):
- Calories: 150
- Protein: 4g
- Fat: 8g
- Carbohydrates: 18g
- Fiber: 4g
- Sugars: 10g

Ingredients (for 4 people):
- 1 tablespoon olive oil
- 1 onion, chopped
- 2 cloves garlic, minced
- 2 cans peeled tomatoes (28 oz each)
- 4 cups low-sodium vegetable broth
- 1/4 cup fresh basil, chopped
- Salt and pepper to taste
- 1/4 cup light cream (optional)

Instructions:
1. In a large pot, heat the olive oil over medium heat. Add the onion and garlic and cook until tender, about 5 minutes.
2. Add the peeled tomatoes with their juice and crush them slightly with a wooden spoon.
3. Pour in the vegetable broth and bring to a boil.
4. Reduce heat and simmer for 20 minutes.
5. Use an immersion blender to puree the soup until smooth.
6. Add fresh basil and light cream if using.
7. Season with salt and pepper to taste.
8. Serve hot.

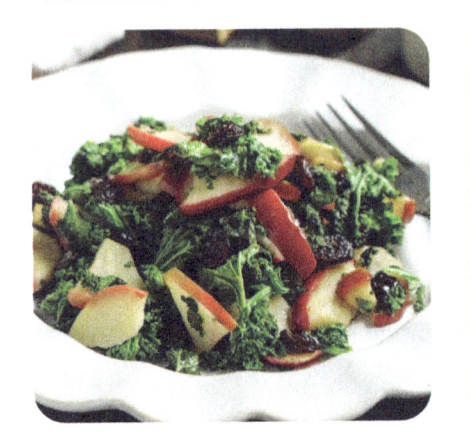

Kale and Apple Salad

NRV (per serving):
- Calories: 220
- Protein: 2g
- Fat: 12g
- Carbohydrates: 30g
- Fiber: 6g
- Sugars: 20g

Ingredients (for 4 people):
- 4 cups shredded kale
- 2 apples, thinly sliced
- 1/4 cup chopped pecans
- 1/4 cup raisins
- 2 tablespoons olive oil
- Juice of 1 lemon
- 1 tablespoon honey
- Salt and pepper to taste

Instructions:
1. In a large bowl, combine the kale, apples, pecans, and raisins.
2. In a small bowl, whisk together the olive oil, lemon juice, honey, salt, and pepper.
3. Pour the dressing over the salad and mix well.
4. Let sit for at least 10 minutes before serving to allow the flavors to meld.
5. Serve as a side dish or main course.

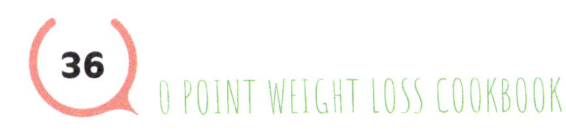

Snacks

Hummus with Crudités

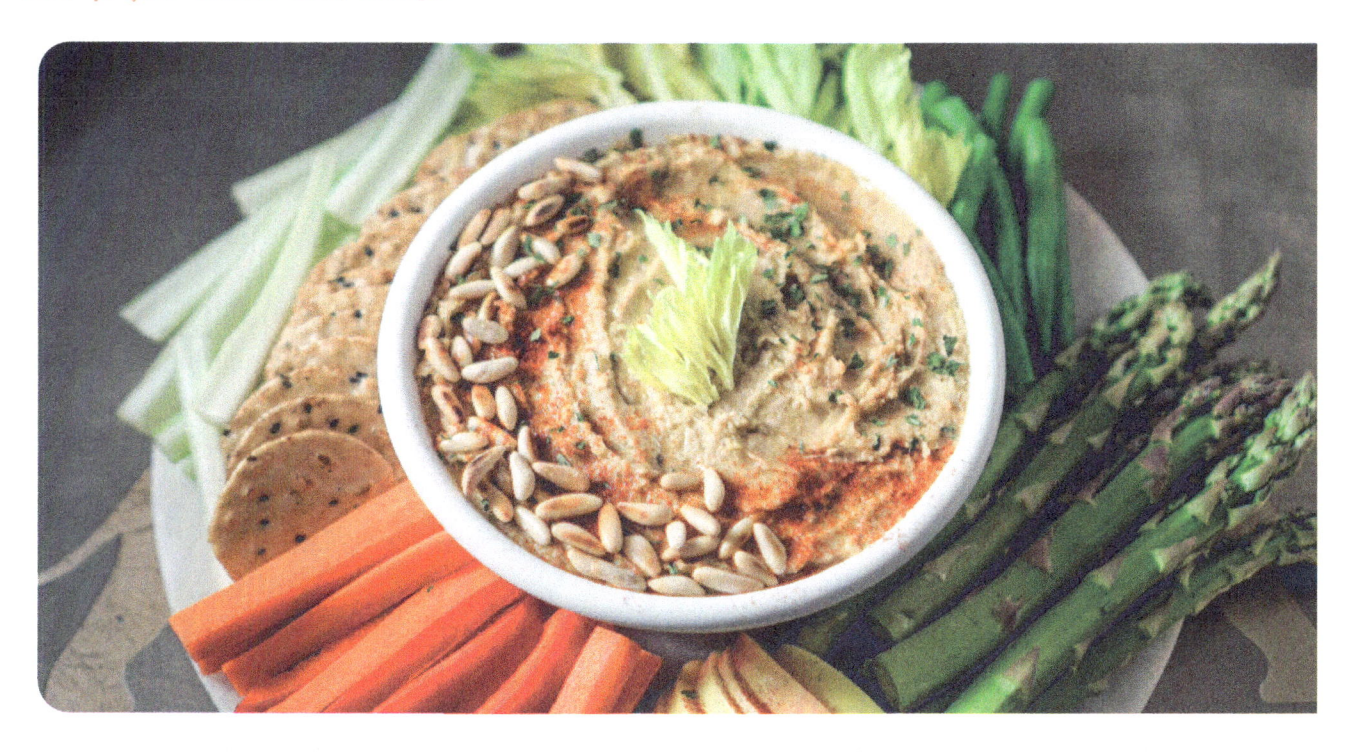

Ingredients (for 4 people):

- 1 can of chickpeas (15 oz), drained and rinsed
- 1/4 cup tahini
- 2 tablespoons lemon juice
- 2 cloves garlic, minced
- 2 tablespoons olive oil
- 1/4 teaspoon ground cumin
- Salt and pepper to taste
- 1/4 cup water (adjust quantity to achieve desired consistency)
- 1 carrot, cut into sticks
- 1 red bell pepper, sliced
- 1 cucumber, sliced
- 1 celery stalk, cut into sticks

Instructions:

1. In a blender or food processor, combine the chickpeas, tahini, lemon juice, garlic, olive oil, and cumin.
2. Blend until smooth, adding water gradually until the desired consistency is reached.
3. Season with salt and pepper to taste.
4. Transfer the hummus to a bowl and serve with the raw vegetables.

NRV (per serving):

- Calories: 200
- Protein: 5g
- Fat: 12g
- Carbohydrates: 18g
- Fiber: 6g
- Sugars: 3g

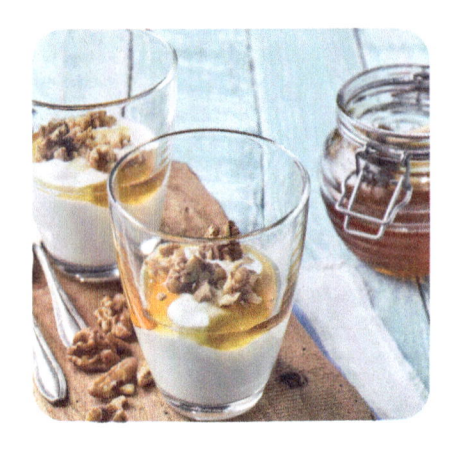

Greek Yogurt with Honey and Nuts

NRV (per serving):
- Calories: 200
- Protein: 15g
- Fat: 8g
- Carbohydrates: 18g
- Fiber: 2g
- Sugars: 12g

Ingredients (for 2 people):
- 1 cup fat-free Greek yogurt
- 2 teaspoons honey
- 1/4 cup chopped nuts

Instructions:
1. Divide the Greek yogurt into two bowls.
2. Drizzle 1 teaspoon of honey over each portion of yogurt.
3. Sprinkle 2 tablespoons of chopped nuts over each portion.
4. Mix well and serve immediately.

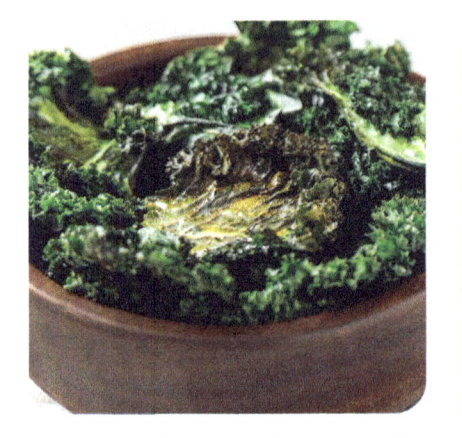

Kale Chips

NRV (per serving):
- Calories: 70
- Protein: 3g
- Fat: 4g
- Carbohydrates: 8g
- Fiber: 2g
- Sugars: 1g

Ingredients (for 2 people):
- 1 bunch kale
- 1 tablespoon olive oil
- 1/2 teaspoon sea salt

Instructions:
1. Preheat the oven to 350°F (175°C).
2. Wash and thoroughly dry the kale, then remove the tough stems and tear the leaves into bite-sized pieces.
3. In a large bowl, toss the kale with olive oil and sea salt.
4. Spread the kale in a single layer on a baking sheet lined with parchment paper.
5. Bake for 10-15 minutes or until the leaves are crispy. Be careful not to burn them.
6. Let cool slightly and serve.

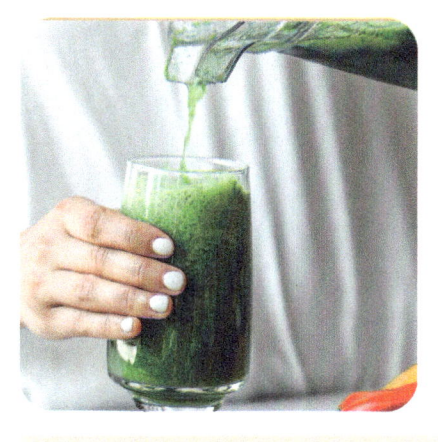

Green Smoothie

NRV (per serving):
- Calories: 180
- Protein: 4g
- Fat: 4g
- Carbohydrates: 36g
- Fiber: 8g
- Sugars: 18g

Ingredients (for 1 person):
- 1 cup fresh spinach
- 1 ripe banana
- 1/2 cup fresh or frozen pineapple
- 1/2 cup unsweetened almond milk
- 1 tablespoon chia seeds (optional)

Instructions:
1. Place the spinach, banana, pineapple, and almond milk in a blender.
2. Blend until smooth and consistent.
3. Add chia seeds if desired and mix well.
4. Pour into a glass and serve immediately.

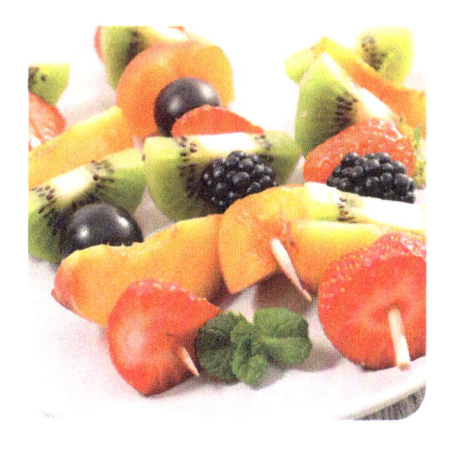

Fruit Skewers

NRV (per serving):
- Calories: 70
- Protein: 1g
- Fat: 0g
- Carbohydrates: 18g
- Fiber: 3g
- Sugars: 12g

Ingredients (for 4 people):
- 1 cup strawberries, halved
- 1 cup pineapple, cubed
- 1 banana, sliced
- 1 kiwi, sliced
- 1 cup seedless grapes

Instructions:
1. Wash and prepare all the fruit.
2. Thread the fruit pieces onto skewers in any order you like.
3. Arrange the skewers on a serving platter.
4. Serve immediately or refrigerate until ready to serve.

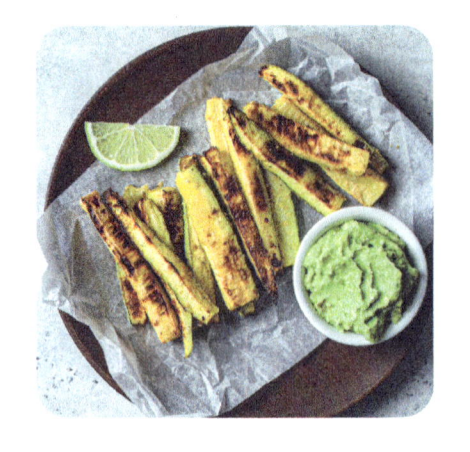

Guacamole with Vegetable Sticks

NRV (per serving):
- Calories: 150
- Protein: 2g
- Fat: 12g
- Carbohydrates: 12g
- Fiber: 6g
- Sugars: 3g

Ingredients (for 4 people):
- 2 ripe avocados
- Juice of 1 lime
- 1/2 cup cherry tomatoes, diced
- 1/4 cup red onion, chopped
- 2 tablespoons fresh cilantro, chopped
- 1/2 teaspoon garlic powder
- Salt and pepper to taste
- 2 carrots, cut into sticks
- 2 celery stalks, cut into sticks
- 1 red bell pepper, sliced

Instructions:
5. In a bowl, mash the avocados with a fork.
6. Add the lime juice, cherry tomatoes, red onion, cilantro, garlic powder, salt, and pepper. Mix well.
7. Transfer the guacamole to a serving bowl.
8. Serve with vegetable sticks.

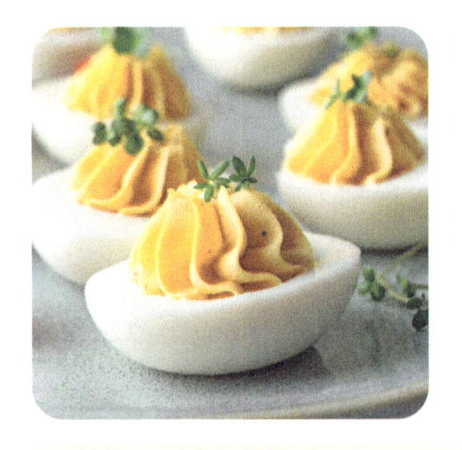

Deviled Eggs

NRV (per serving):
- Calories: 80
- Protein: 6g
- Fat: 5g
- Carbohydrates: 1g
- Fiber: 0g
- Sugars: 1g

Ingredients (for 4 people):
- 4 hard-boiled eggs
- 2 tablespoons fat-free Greek yogurt
- 1 teaspoon Dijon mustard
- 1/4 teaspoon paprika
- Salt and pepper to taste
- Paprika for garnish

Instructions:
1. Cut the hard-boiled eggs in half lengthwise. Remove the yolks and place them in a bowl.
2. Mash the yolks with a fork and add the Greek yogurt, Dijon mustard, paprika, salt, and pepper. Mix well.
3. Fill the egg whites with the yolk mixture.
4. Sprinkle with paprika for garnish.
5. Serve immediately or refrigerate until ready to serve.

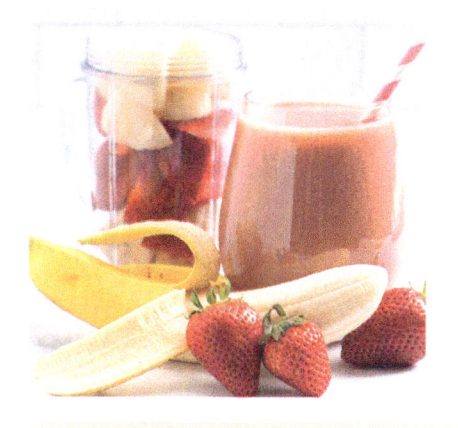

Strawberry Banana Smoothie

NRV (per serving):
- Calories: 200
- Protein: 10g
- Fat: 2g
- Carbohydrates: 38g
- Fiber: 5g
- Sugars: 20g

Ingredients (for 1 person):
- 1 cup fresh or frozen strawberries
- 1 ripe banana
- 1/2 cup fat-free Greek yogurt
- 1/2 cup unsweetened almond milk
- 1 teaspoon honey (optional)

Instructions:
1. Place the strawberries, banana, Greek yogurt, and almond milk in a blender.
2. Blend until smooth and consistent.
3. Add honey if desired and blend again.
4. Pour into a glass and serve immediately.

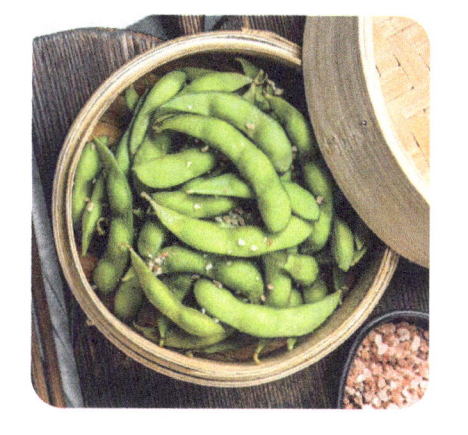

Steamed Edamame with Sea Salt

NRV (per serving):
- Calories: 120
- Protein: 11g
- Fat: 5g
- Carbohydrates: 10g
- Fiber: 4g
- Sugars: 1g

Ingredients (for 4 people):
- 2 cups frozen edamame
- 1/2 teaspoon sea salt

Instructions:
1. Bring a pot of water to a boil.
2. Add the frozen edamame and cook for 4-5 minutes or until tender.
3. Drain and transfer the edamame to a bowl.
4. Sprinkle with sea salt and mix well.
5. Serve immediately.

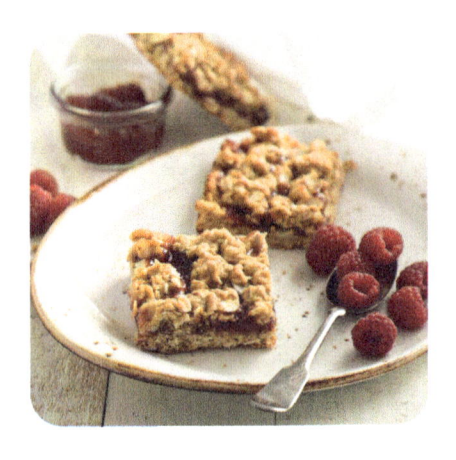

Blueberry Oat Bars

NRV (per bar):
- Calories: 200
- Protein: 5g
- Fat: 9g
- Carbohydrates: 28g
- Fiber: 4g
- Sugars: 12g

Ingredients (for 8 bars):
- 2 cups rolled oats
- 1 cup fresh or frozen blueberries
- 1/2 cup chopped almonds
- 1/4 cup honey
- 1/4 cup almond butter
- 1 teaspoon vanilla extract
- 1/4 teaspoon salt

Instructions:
1. Preheat the oven to 350°F (175°C). Line a baking dish with parchment paper.
2. In a large bowl, mix the rolled oats, blueberries, and almonds.
3. In a saucepan over medium heat, melt the honey and almond butter until smooth.
4. Add the vanilla extract and salt to the honey and almond butter mixture.
5. Pour the liquid mixture over the dry ingredients and mix well until everything is well combined.
6. Transfer the mixture to the prepared baking dish and press it firmly.
7. Bake in the oven for 20-25 minutes or until the bars are golden.
8. Let cool completely before cutting into bars.
9. Store in an airtight container.

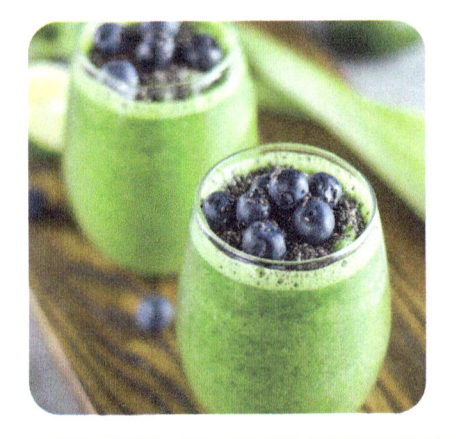

Blueberry Spinach Smoothie

NRV (per serving):
- Calories: 180
- Protein: 4g
- Fat: 3g
- Carbohydrates: 38g
- Fiber: 8g
- Sugars: 20g

Ingredients (for 1 person):
- 1 cup fresh or frozen blueberries
- 1 cup fresh spinach
- 1 ripe banana
- 1/2 cup unsweetened almond milk
- 1 tablespoon flax seeds (optional)

Instructions:
1. Place the blueberries, spinach, banana, and almond milk in a blender.
2. Blend until smooth and consistent.
3. Add flax seeds if desired and mix well.
4. Pour into a glass and serve immediately.

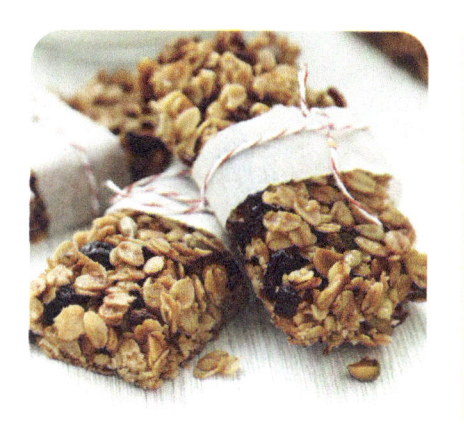

Cereal and Nut Bars

NRV (per bar):
- Calories: 210
- Protein: 5g
- Fat: 9g
- Carbohydrates: 30g
- Fiber: 4g
- Sugars: 14g

Ingredients (for 8 bars):
- 1 1/2 cups rolled oats
- 1/2 cup chopped almonds
- 1/2 cup dried cranberries
- 1/4 cup pumpkin seeds
- 1/4 cup honey
- 1/4 cup almond butter
- 1 teaspoon vanilla extract
- 1/4 teaspoon salt

Instructions:
1. Preheat the oven to 350°F (175°C). Line a baking dish with parchment paper.
2. In a large bowl, mix the rolled oats, almonds, cranberries, and pumpkin seeds.
3. In a saucepan over medium heat, melt the honey and almond butter until smooth.
4. Add the vanilla extract and salt to the honey and almond butter mixture.
5. Pour the liquid mixture over the dry ingredients and mix well until everything is well combined.
6. Transfer the mixture to the prepared baking dish and press it firmly.
7. Bake in the oven for 20-25 minutes or until the bars are golden.
8. Let cool completely before cutting into bars.
9. Store in an airtight container.

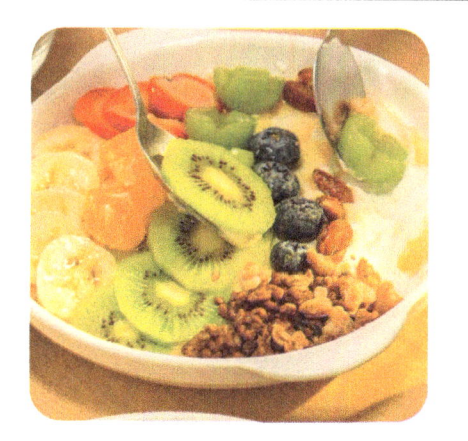

Mixed Fruit with Greek Yogurt

NRV (per serving):
- Calories: 180
- Protein: 12g
- Fat: 0g
- Carbohydrates: 35g
- Fiber: 5g
- Sugars: 20g

Ingredients (for 2 people):
- 1 cup strawberries, halved
- 1 cup blueberries
- 1 banana, sliced
- 1 cup fat-free Greek yogurt
- 2 teaspoons honey (optional)

Instructions:
1. In a large bowl, mix the strawberries, blueberries, and banana.
2. Divide the mixed fruit into two bowls.
3. Add 1/2 cup of Greek yogurt on top of the fruit in each bowl.
4. Drizzle 1 teaspoon of honey over the yogurt if desired.
5. Mix gently and serve immediately.

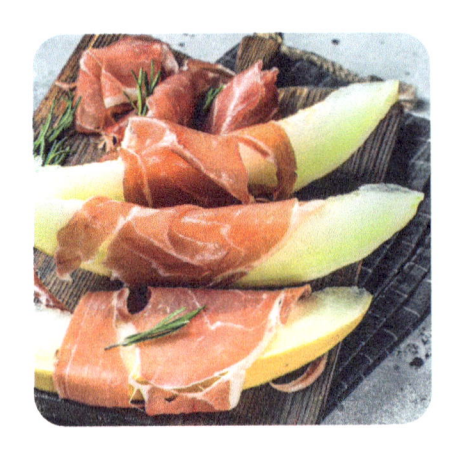

Melon Wrapped in Prosciutto

NRV (per serving):
- Calories: 100
- Protein: 6g
- Fat: 3g
- Carbohydrates: 14g
- Fiber: 1g
- Sugars: 13g

Ingredients (for 4 people):
- 1 cantaloupe melon, sliced
- 8 slices prosciutto

Instructions:
1. Wrap each melon slice with a slice of prosciutto.
2. Arrange on a serving platter.
3. Serve immediately.

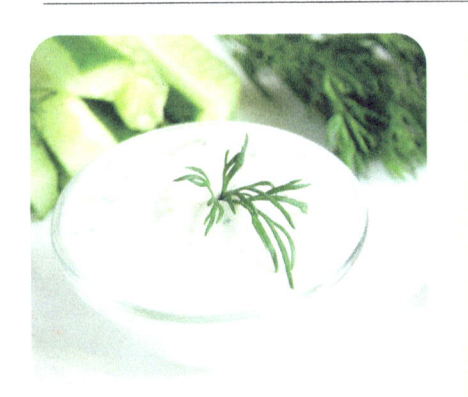

Cucumber Sticks with Yogurt Dip

NRV (per serving):
- Calories: 60
- Protein: 5g
- Fat: 0g
- Carbohydrates: 10g
- Fiber: 2g
- Sugars: 6g

Ingredients (for 2 people):
- 1 cucumber, cut into sticks
- 1/2 cup fat-free Greek yogurt
- 1 teaspoon lemon juice
- 1 tablespoon fresh dill, chopped
- Salt and pepper to taste

Instructions:
1. In a small bowl, mix the Greek yogurt, lemon juice, dill, salt, and pepper.
2. Arrange the cucumber sticks on a serving platter.
3. Serve the cucumber sticks with the yogurt dip.

Dinners

Baked Salmon with Asparagus

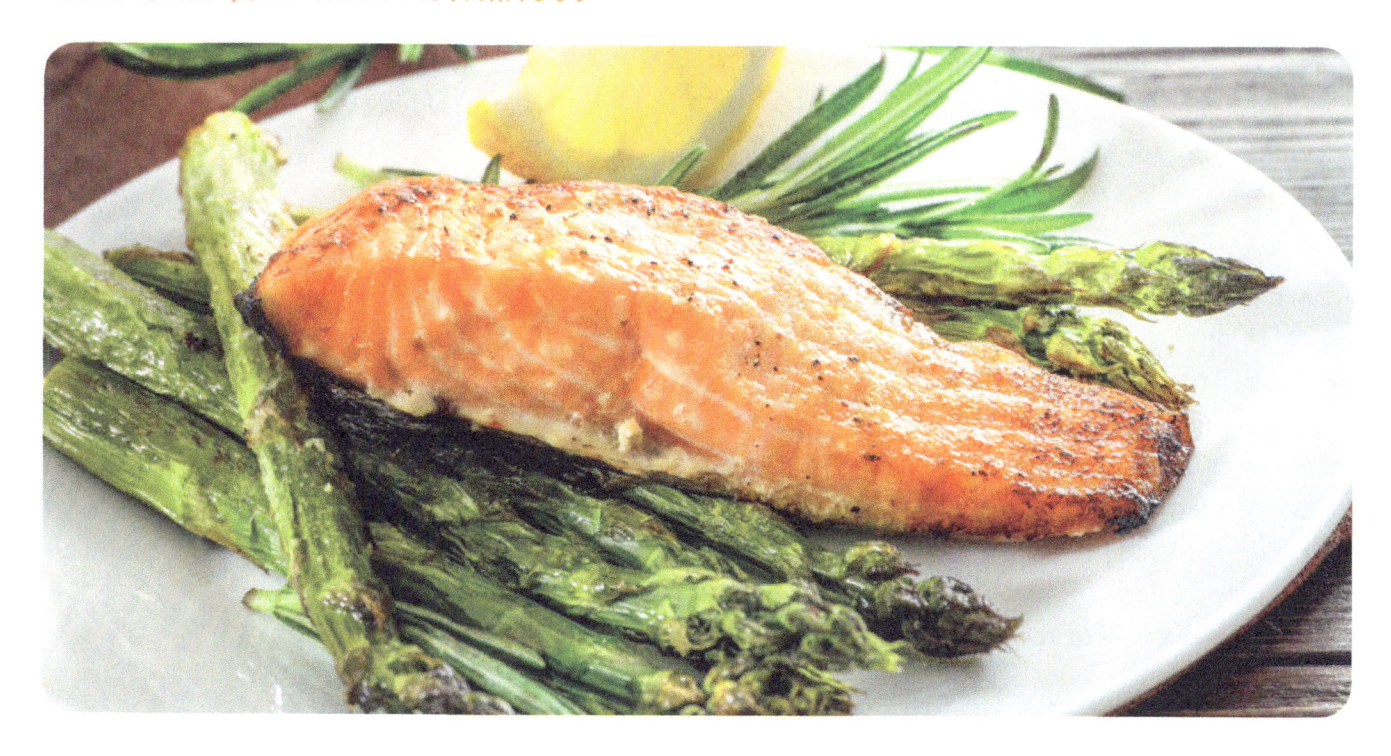

Ingredients (for 2 people):

- 2 salmon fillets (about 6 oz each)
- 1 bunch of asparagus, trimmed and cut into pieces
- 1 lemon, sliced
- 2 cloves garlic, minced
- 2 tablespoons olive oil
- Salt and pepper to taste
- 1 tablespoon fresh parsley, chopped (optional)

Instructions:

1. Preheat the oven to 400°F (200°C).
2. Arrange the salmon fillets on a baking sheet lined with parchment paper. Spread the asparagus around the salmon.
3. Drizzle the salmon and asparagus with olive oil and sprinkle with minced garlic, salt, and pepper.
4. Place the lemon slices on top of the salmon and asparagus.
5. Bake in the oven for 15-20 minutes or until the salmon is cooked through and the asparagus is tender.
6. Garnish with fresh parsley if desired and serve hot.

NRV (per serving):

- Calories: 350
- Protein: 30g
- Fat: 20g
- Carbohydrates: 10g
- Fiber: 4g
- Sugars: 2g

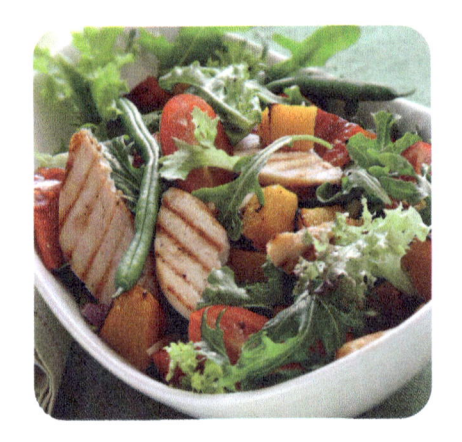

Grilled Chicken with Mixed Vegetables

NRV (per serving):
- Calories: 400
- Protein: 35g
- Fat: 25g
- Carbohydrates: 12g
- Fiber: 4g
- Sugars: 6g

Ingredients (for 2 people):
- 2 skinless chicken breasts
- 1 zucchini, sliced
- 1 red bell pepper, sliced
- 1 red onion, sliced
- 1/4 cup olive oil
- Juice of 1 lemon
- 2 cloves garlic, minced
- 1 teaspoon dried oregano
- Salt and pepper to taste

Instructions:
1. In a bowl, mix the olive oil, lemon juice, minced garlic, oregano, salt, and pepper.
2. Add the chicken breasts to the marinade and let sit for at least 30 minutes.
3. Preheat a grill to medium-high heat. Grill the chicken for 6-7 minutes per side or until fully cooked.
4. Meanwhile, grill the vegetables until tender and slightly charred.
5. Serve the grilled chicken with the mixed vegetables.

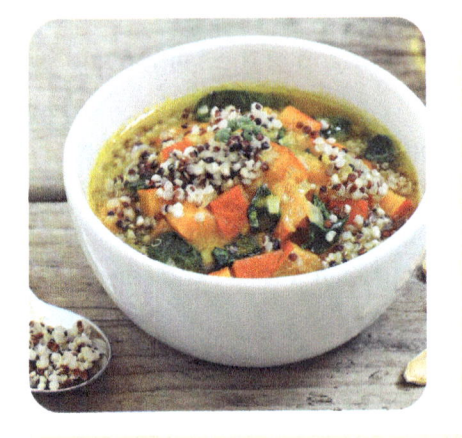

Vegetable Soup with Quinoa

NRV (per serving):
- Calories: 250
- Protein: 8g
- Fat: 8g
- Carbohydrates: 38g
- Fiber: 6g
- Sugars: 7g

Ingredients (for 4 people):
- 1 cup quinoa
- 2 tablespoons olive oil
- 1 onion, chopped
- 2 carrots, sliced
- 2 celery stalks, sliced
- 1 zucchini, diced
- 1 can diced tomatoes (15 oz)
- 6 cups low-sodium vegetable broth
- 1 teaspoon dried thyme
- 1 bay leaf
- Salt and pepper to taste
- Fresh parsley, chopped (optional)

Instructions:
1. Rinse the quinoa under cold running water.
2. In a large pot, heat the olive oil over medium heat. Add the onion, carrots, and celery and cook until tender, about 5 minutes.
3. Add the zucchini and cook for another 2 minutes.
4. Add the diced tomatoes, vegetable broth, quinoa, thyme, and bay leaf.
5. Bring to a boil, then reduce heat and simmer for 20-25 minutes or until the quinoa is tender.
6. Remove the bay leaf and season with salt and pepper to taste.
7. Serve hot, garnished with fresh parsley if desired.

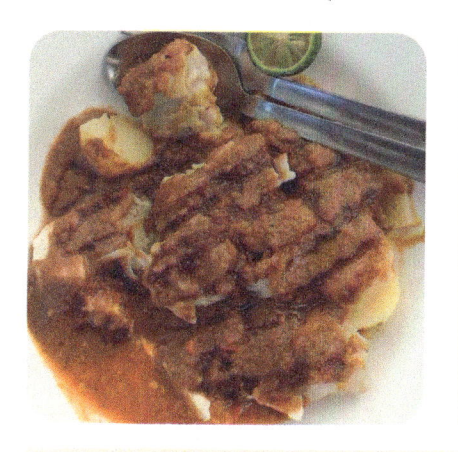

Grilled Tofu with Peanut Sauce

NRV (per serving):
- Calories: 350
- Protein: 18g
- Fat: 25g
- Carbohydrates: 20g
- Fiber: 4g
- Sugars: 8g

Ingredients (for 2 people):
- 1 block tofu (about 14 oz), sliced
- 2 tablespoons sesame oil
- 2 tablespoons low-sodium soy sauce
- 1 tablespoon lime juice
- 1 teaspoon fresh ginger, grated
- 1/4 cup peanut butter
- 2 tablespoons water
- 1 tablespoon rice vinegar
- 1 tablespoon honey
- 1 clove garlic, minced
- 1/4 teaspoon cayenne pepper (optional)
- Fresh cilantro, chopped (optional)

Instructions:
1. In a bowl, mix the sesame oil, soy sauce, lime juice, and ginger.
2. Add the tofu to the marinade and let sit for at least 30 minutes.
3. Preheat a grill to medium-high heat. Grill the tofu for 4-5 minutes per side or until well marked.
4. Meanwhile, in a small bowl, mix the peanut butter, water, rice vinegar, honey, garlic, and cayenne pepper until smooth.
5. Serve the grilled tofu with the peanut sauce and garnish with fresh cilantro if desired.

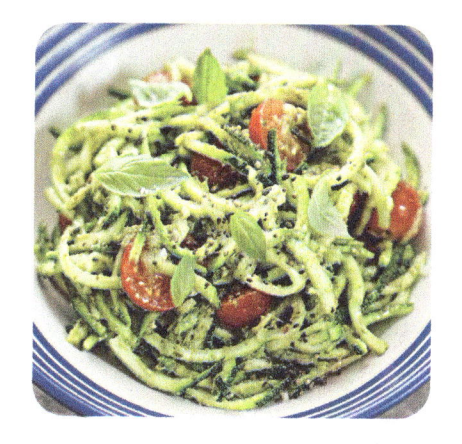

Zucchini Noodles with Cherry Tomatoes and Basil

NRV (per serving):
- Calories: 180
- Protein: 4g
- Fat: 14g
- Carbohydrates: 14g
- Fiber: 5g
- Sugars: 8g

Ingredients (for 2 people):
- 4 medium zucchinis, spiralized
- 2 tablespoons olive oil
- 1 pint cherry tomatoes, halved
- 2 cloves garlic, minced
- 1/4 cup fresh basil, chopped
- Salt and pepper to taste
- 1/4 cup grated Parmesan cheese (optional)

Instructions:
1. Heat the olive oil in a large skillet over medium heat. Add the garlic and cook for 1-2 minutes until fragrant.
2. Add the cherry tomatoes and cook for 5-7 minutes until they start to break down.
3. Add the zucchini noodles to the skillet and cook for another 3-5 minutes, stirring frequently, until tender.
4. Season with salt and pepper to taste.
5. Remove from heat and add the fresh basil.
6. Serve immediately, garnished with grated Parmesan cheese if desired.

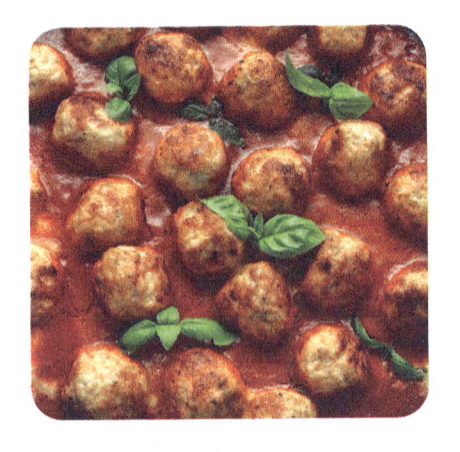

Baked Turkey Meatballs with Tomato Sauce

NRV (per serving):
- Calories: 250
- Protein: 25g
- Fat: 12g
- Carbohydrates: 12g
- Fiber: 3g
- Sugars: 5g

Ingredients (for 4 people):
- 1 lb ground turkey
- 1 egg
- 1/4 cup whole-wheat breadcrumbs
- 1/4 cup grated Parmesan cheese
- 2 cloves garlic, minced
- 1 teaspoon dried oregano
- 1 teaspoon dried basil
- Salt and pepper to taste
- 2 cups low-sodium tomato sauce
- 1 tablespoon olive oil

Instructions:
1. Preheat the oven to 375°F (190°C). Lightly grease a baking sheet with olive oil.
2. In a large bowl, mix the ground turkey, egg, breadcrumbs, Parmesan cheese, garlic, oregano, basil, salt, and pepper.
3. Form the mixture into meatballs and place them on the prepared baking sheet.
4. Bake in the oven for 20-25 minutes or until the meatballs are golden and fully cooked.
5. Meanwhile, heat the tomato sauce in a saucepan over medium heat.
6. When the meatballs are cooked, transfer them to the tomato sauce and cook for another 5 minutes.
7. Serve hot, garnished with fresh basil if desired.

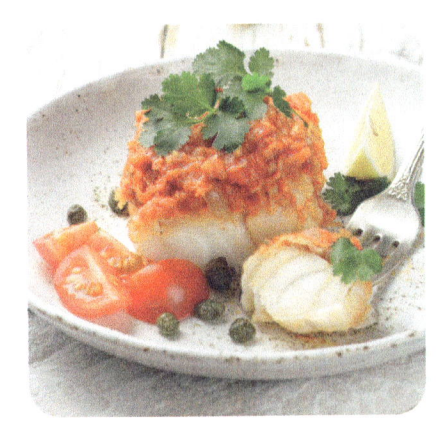

Lemon Caper Cod Fillets

NRV (per serving):
- Calories: 220
- Protein: 28g
- Fat: 10g
- Carbohydrates: 4g
- Fiber: 1g
- Sugars: 1g

Ingredients (for 2 people):
- 2 cod fillets (about 6 oz each)
- 2 tablespoons olive oil
- Juice of 1 lemon
- 1/4 cup capers, rinsed
- 2 cloves garlic, minced
- Salt and pepper to taste
- Fresh parsley, chopped (optional)

Instructions:
1. Heat the olive oil in a large skillet over medium-high heat.
2. Season the cod fillets with salt and pepper.
3. Add the cod fillets to the skillet and cook for 3-4 minutes per side or until golden and cooked through.
4. Remove the cod from the skillet and set aside.
5. In the same skillet, add the garlic and capers and cook for 1-2 minutes until fragrant.
6. Add the lemon juice and stir well.
7. Return the cod fillets to the skillet and cook for another 2 minutes, basting with the sauce.
8. Serve hot, garnished with fresh parsley if desired.

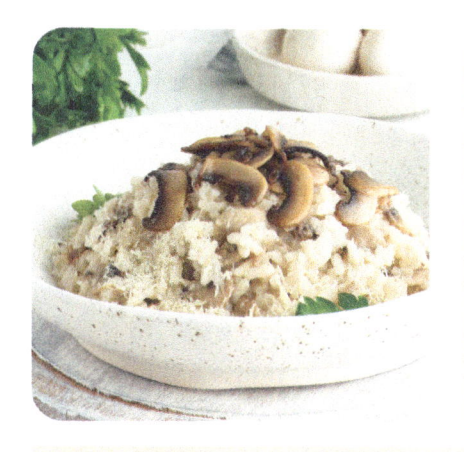

Mushroom Risotto

NRV (per serving):
- Calories: 300
- Protein: 8g
- Fat: 12g
- Carbohydrates: 38g
- Fiber: 3g
- Sugars: 2g

Ingredients (for 4 people):
- 1 cup arborio rice
- 4 cups low-sodium vegetable broth
- 1 cup dried porcini mushrooms
- 1 onion, chopped
- 2 cloves garlic, minced
- 1/2 cup dry white wine
- 2 tablespoons olive oil
- 1/4 cup grated Parmesan cheese
- 1 tablespoon butter (optional)
- Salt and pepper to taste
- Fresh parsley, chopped (optional)

Instructions:
1. Bring the broth to a simmer in a pot and keep warm.
2. In a bowl, cover the dried porcini mushrooms with hot water and let soak for 20 minutes. Drain, reserving the soaking liquid, and chop the mushrooms.
3. In a large skillet, heat the olive oil over medium heat. Add the onion and garlic and cook until tender, about 5 minutes.
4. Add the chopped mushrooms and cook for another 2 minutes.
5. Add the arborio rice and cook, stirring constantly, until the grains are translucent, about 2 minutes.
6. Add the white wine and cook until evaporated.
7. Add a ladleful of hot broth to the rice and cook, stirring continuously, until the liquid is absorbed. Repeat, adding broth one ladle at a time, until the rice is creamy and cooked al dente, about 18-20 minutes.
8. Add the reserved mushroom soaking liquid for extra flavor during the cooking process.
9. Remove from heat and stir in the Parmesan cheese and butter if using. Season with salt and pepper to taste.
10. Serve hot, garnished with fresh parsley if desired.

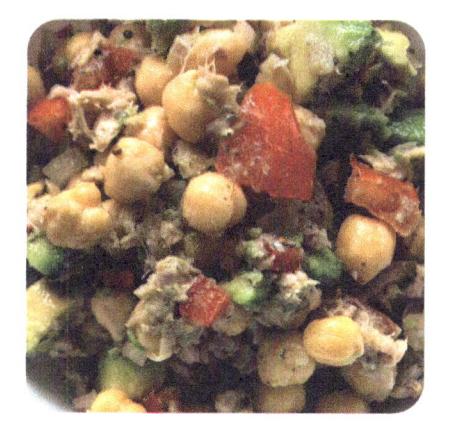

Chickpea and Tuna Salad

NRV (per serving):
- Calories: 250
- Protein: 20g
- Fat: 12g
- Carbohydrates: 18g
- Fiber: 6g
- Sugars: 3g

Ingredients (for 4 people):
- 1 can chickpeas (15 oz), drained and rinsed
- 2 cans tuna in water (5 oz each), drained
- 1/2 cup cherry tomatoes, halved
- 1/4 cup red onion, chopped
- 1/4 cup black olives, sliced
- 2 tablespoons capers, drained
- 2 tablespoons olive oil
- Juice of 1 lemon
- Salt and pepper to taste
- Fresh parsley, chopped (optional)

Instructions:
1. In a large bowl, combine the chickpeas, tuna, cherry tomatoes, red onion, black olives, and capers.
2. In a small bowl, whisk together the olive oil and lemon juice.
3. Pour the dressing over the salad and toss gently to combine.
4. Season with salt and pepper to taste.
5. Serve immediately or refrigerate until ready to serve. Garnish with fresh parsley if desired.

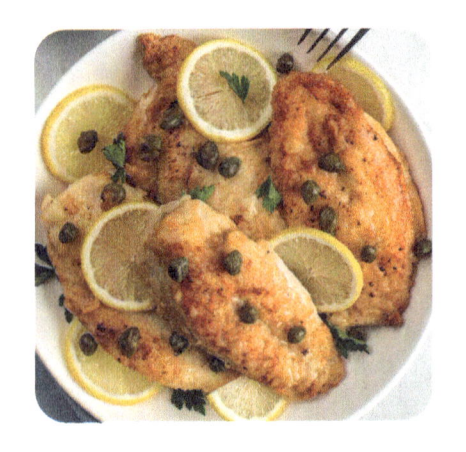

Lemon Caper Chicken

NRV (per serving):
- Calories: 270
- Protein: 26g
- Fat: 12g
- Carbohydrates: 12g
- Fiber: 1g
- Sugars: 1g

Ingredients (for 4 people):
- 1 lb skinless chicken breasts, halved
- 2 tablespoons olive oil
- 1/4 cup whole-wheat flour
- Juice of 2 lemons
- 1/4 cup capers, rinsed
- 1/2 cup low-sodium chicken broth
- 2 cloves garlic, minced
- Salt and pepper to taste
- Fresh parsley, chopped (optional)

Instructions:
1. Lightly coat the chicken breasts with flour.
2. In a large skillet, heat the olive oil over medium-high heat.
3. Add the chicken breasts and cook for 4-5 minutes per side or until golden and cooked through.
4. Remove the chicken from the skillet and set aside.
5. In the same skillet, add the minced garlic and cook for 1-2 minutes until fragrant.
6. Add the lemon juice, capers, and chicken broth. Bring to a simmer and cook for 3-4 minutes until the sauce slightly reduces.
7. Return the chicken to the skillet and cook for another 2 minutes, basting with the sauce.
8. Season with salt and pepper to taste.
9. Serve hot, garnished with fresh parsley if desired.

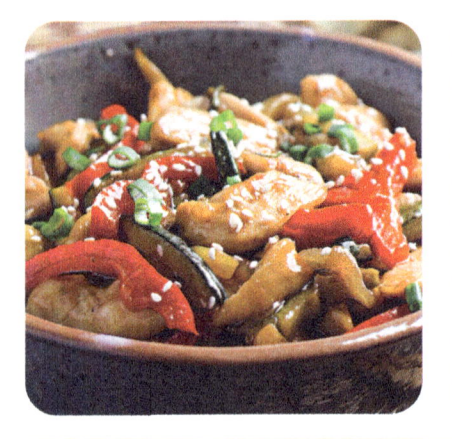

Sesame Chicken with Zucchini

NRV (per serving):
- Calories: 280
- Protein: 25g
- Fat: 12g
- Carbohydrates: 15g
- Fiber: 2g
- Sugars: 10g

Ingredients (for 4 people):
- 1 lb skinless chicken breasts, cubed
- 2 zucchinis, sliced
- 2 tablespoons sesame oil
- 2 cloves garlic, minced
- 1/4 cup low-sodium soy sauce
- 2 tablespoons honey
- 1 tablespoon sesame seeds
- 1/4 cup green onions, chopped
- Salt and pepper to taste

Instructions:
1. In a large skillet, heat the sesame oil over medium-high heat.
2. Add the chicken and cook for 6-7 minutes until golden and cooked through.
3. Add the minced garlic and cook for 1 minute.
4. Add the zucchini and cook for another 5 minutes until tender.
5. In a bowl, mix the soy sauce and honey. Pour the mixture into the skillet and stir well to coat the chicken and zucchini.
6. Cook for another 2 minutes until the sauce thickens.
7. Season with salt and pepper to taste.
8. Sprinkle with sesame seeds and chopped green onions before serving.

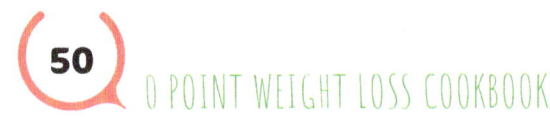

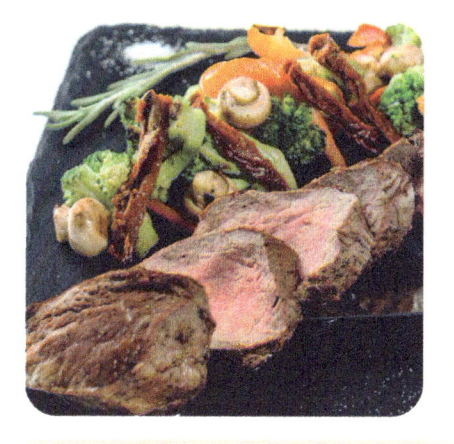

Grilled Pork Tenderloin with Vegetables

NRV (per serving):
- Calories: 300
- Protein: 25g
- Fat: 16g
- Carbohydrates: 12g
- Fiber: 3g
- Sugars: 6g

Ingredients (for 4 people):
- 1 lb pork tenderloin
- 1 red bell pepper, sliced
- 1 yellow bell pepper, sliced
- 1 zucchini, sliced
- 1 red onion, cut into wedges
- 2 tablespoons olive oil
- 2 tablespoons low-sodium soy sauce
- 1 tablespoon balsamic vinegar
- 2 cloves garlic, minced
- Salt and pepper to taste
- Fresh rosemary, chopped (optional)

Instructions:
1. In a bowl, mix the olive oil, soy sauce, balsamic vinegar, garlic, salt, and pepper.
2. Place the pork tenderloin in a bowl or zip-top bag and pour half of the marinade over it. Let marinate for at least 30 minutes.
3. Preheat the grill to medium-high heat.
4. Grill the pork tenderloin for 15-20 minutes, turning occasionally, until cooked through. Let rest for 5 minutes before slicing.
5. Meanwhile, toss the vegetables with the remaining marinade.
6. Grill the vegetables until tender and slightly charred.
7. Serve the sliced pork tenderloin with the grilled vegetables, garnished with fresh rosemary if desired.

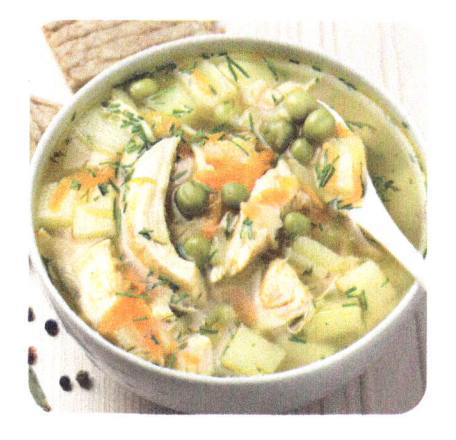

Chicken and Vegetable Soup

NRV (per serving):
- Calories: 200
- Protein: 25g
- Fat: 5g
- Carbohydrates: 12g
- Fiber: 3g
- Sugars: 4g

Ingredients (for 4 people):
- 1 lb skinless chicken breasts
- 6 cups low-sodium chicken broth
- 2 carrots, sliced
- 2 celery stalks, sliced
- 1 onion, chopped
- 2 cloves garlic, minced
- 1 zucchini, diced
- 1 cup fresh spinach
- 1 teaspoon dried thyme
- 1 bay leaf
- Salt and pepper to taste
- Fresh parsley, chopped (optional)

Instructions:
1. In a large pot, bring the chicken broth to a boil. Add the chicken breasts and cook for 15-20 minutes or until cooked through. Remove the chicken from the broth and let cool slightly, then shred.
2. In the same pot, add the carrots, celery, onion, and garlic. Cook for 5 minutes until the vegetables are tender.
3. Add the zucchini, thyme, and bay leaf. Cook for another 10 minutes.
4. Return the shredded chicken to the pot and add the fresh spinach. Cook until the spinach is wilted.
5. Season with salt and pepper to taste.
6. Serve hot, garnished with fresh parsley if desired.

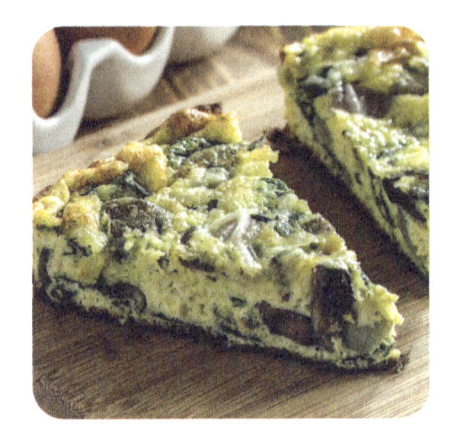

Spinach and Mushroom Frittata

NRV (per serving):
- Calories: 250
- Protein: 18g
- Fat: 18g
- Carbohydrates: 5g
- Fiber: 1g
- Sugars: 2g

Ingredients (for 4 people):
- 8 eggs
- 1/4 cup unsweetened almond milk
- 1 cup mushrooms, sliced
- 1 cup fresh spinach
- 1/4 cup red onion, chopped
- 2 tablespoons olive oil
- Salt and pepper to taste
- 1/4 cup crumbled feta cheese (optional)

Instructions:
1. Preheat the oven to 375°F (190°C).
2. In a large skillet, heat 1 tablespoon olive oil over medium heat. Add the red onion and mushrooms and cook until tender, about 5 minutes.
3. Add the spinach and cook until wilted. Season with salt and pepper.
4. In a large bowl, whisk the eggs with the almond milk, salt, and pepper.
5. Add the cooked vegetables to the egg mixture and mix well.
6. In the same skillet, heat the remaining olive oil over medium heat. Pour the egg and vegetable mixture into the skillet.
7. Cook for 5 minutes, then transfer the skillet to the oven and bake for another 10-15 minutes or until the frittata is fully cooked.
8. If desired, sprinkle the frittata with crumbled feta cheese before serving.

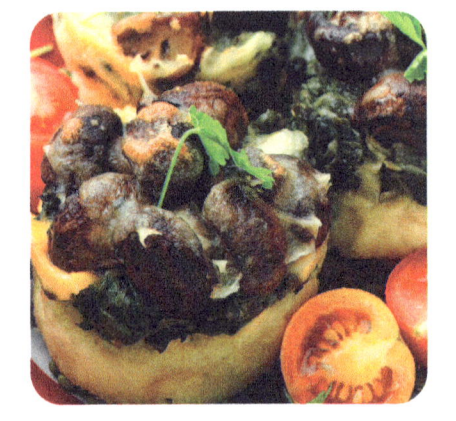

Polenta with Mushrooms and Spinach

NRV (per serving):
- Calories: 300
- Protein: 10g
- Fat: 14g
- Carbohydrates: 38g
- Fiber: 4g
- Sugars: 3g

Ingredients (for 4 people):
- 1 cup polenta
- 4 cups water
- 1/4 cup grated Parmesan cheese
- 1 tablespoon butter
- 2 tablespoons olive oil
- 1 onion, chopped
- 2 cups mushrooms, sliced
- 2 cups fresh spinach
- 2 cloves garlic, minced
- Salt and pepper to taste

Instructions:
1. Bring the water to a boil in a large pot. Gradually add the polenta, stirring continuously.
2. Reduce heat and simmer, stirring frequently, for 30-40 minutes until the polenta is thick and creamy.
3. Remove from heat and stir in the Parmesan cheese and butter. Season with salt and pepper.
4. Meanwhile, in a large skillet, heat the olive oil over medium heat. Add the onion and garlic and cook until tender, about 5 minutes.
5. Add the mushrooms and cook until golden, about 8-10 minutes.
6. Add the spinach and cook until wilted.
7. Season with salt and pepper to taste.
8. Serve the polenta hot, topped with the mushroom and spinach mixture.

Desserts

Avocado Chocolate Mousse

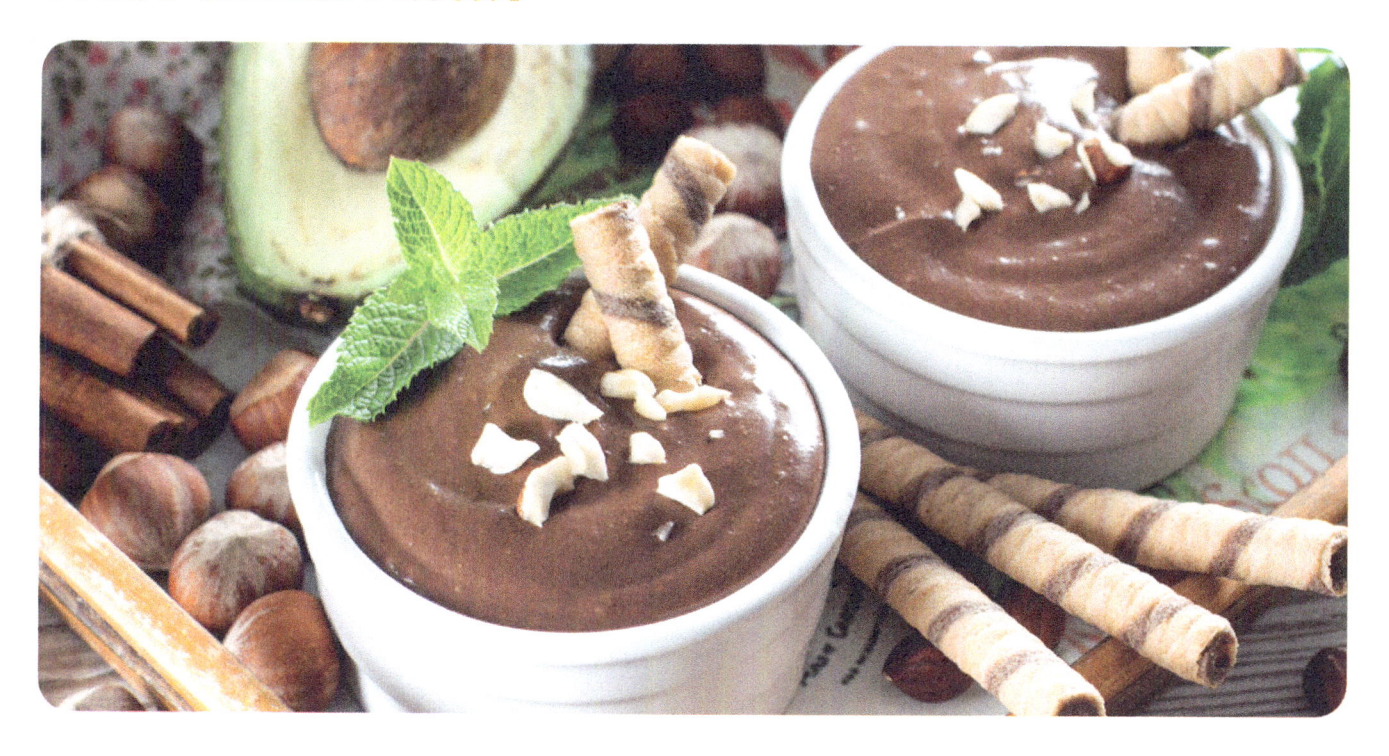

Ingredients (for 4 people):

- 2 ripe avocados
- 1/4 cup unsweetened cocoa powder
- 1/4 cup unsweetened almond milk
- 1/4 cup maple syrup
- 1 teaspoon vanilla extract
- Pinch of salt
- Fresh berries for garnish (optional)

Instructions:

1. In a blender, combine the avocados, cocoa powder, almond milk, maple syrup, vanilla extract, and salt.
2. Blend until smooth and creamy.
3. Divide the mousse into four small bowls.
4. Garnish with fresh berries if desired.
5. Refrigerate for at least 30 minutes before serving.

NRV (per serving):

- Calories: 180
- Protein: 2g
- Fat: 13g
- Carbohydrates: 18g
- Fiber: 6g
- Sugars: 8g

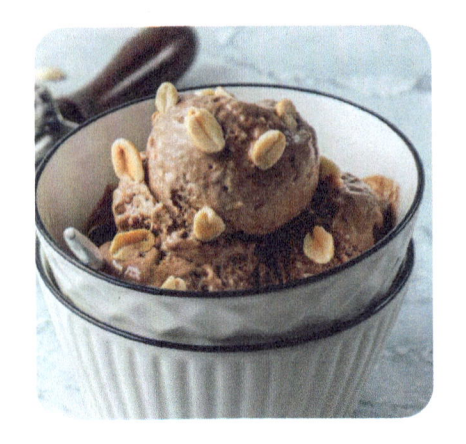

Banana Peanut Butter Ice Cream

NRV (per serving):
- Calories: 150
- Protein: 3g
- Fat: 5g
- Carbohydrates: 28g
- Fiber: 4g
- Sugars: 15g

Ingredients (for 4 people):
- 4 ripe bananas, sliced and frozen
- 2 tablespoons peanut butter
- 1 teaspoon vanilla extract
- 1/4 cup unsweetened almond milk (if needed)

Instructions:
1. Place the frozen bananas in a blender and blend until creamy, adding almond milk if needed.
2. Add the peanut butter and vanilla extract and blend until smooth.
3. Divide the ice cream into four bowls.
4. Serve immediately or store in the freezer until ready to serve.

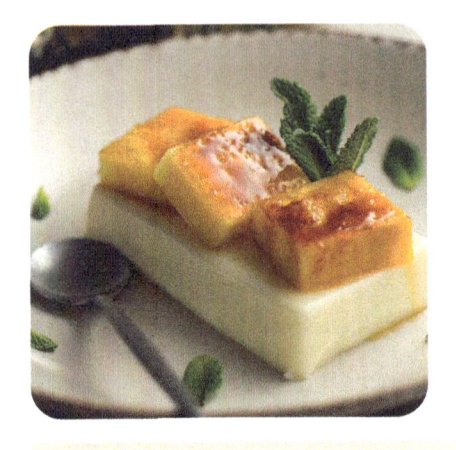

Coconut Panna Cotta

NRV (per serving):
- Calories: 140
- Protein: 2g
- Fat: 10g
- Carbohydrates: 10g
- Fiber: 1g
- Sugars: 8g

Ingredients (for 4 people):
- 1 can light coconut milk (13.5 oz)
- 2 tablespoons maple syrup
- 1 teaspoon vanilla extract
- 1 tablespoon gelatin powder
- 1/4 cup cold water
- Fresh fruit for garnish (optional)

Instructions:
1. In a small bowl, combine the gelatin and cold water. Let sit for 5 minutes.
2. In a saucepan, heat the coconut milk, maple syrup, and vanilla extract over medium heat until warm but not boiling.
3. Add the gelatin mixture and stir until completely dissolved.
4. Pour the mixture into four molds and let cool to room temperature.
5. Cover and refrigerate for at least 4 hours or until set.
6. Garnish with fresh fruit if desired and serve.

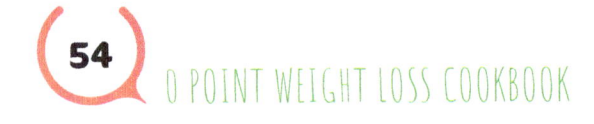

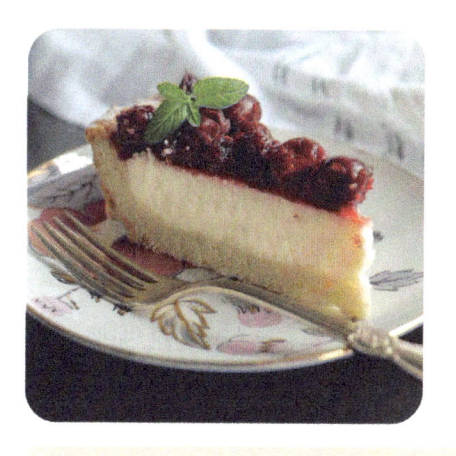

Berry Cheesecake

NRV (per serving):
- Calories: 180
- Protein: 10g
- Fat: 2g
- Carbohydrates: 30g
- Fiber: 3g
- Sugars: 20g

Ingredients (for 6 people):
- 1 cup fat-free ricotta cheese
- 1 cup fat-free Greek yogurt
- 1/4 cup honey
- 1 teaspoon vanilla extract
- 1 cup mixed berries (blueberries, strawberries, raspberries)
- 6 whole-wheat biscuits, crumbled

Instructions:
1. In a bowl, mix the ricotta cheese, Greek yogurt, honey, and vanilla extract until smooth.
2. Divide the cheese mixture into six glasses or bowls.
3. Add a layer of mixed berries on top of the cheese mixture.
4. Sprinkle with crumbled biscuits.
5. Refrigerate for at least 1 hour before serving.

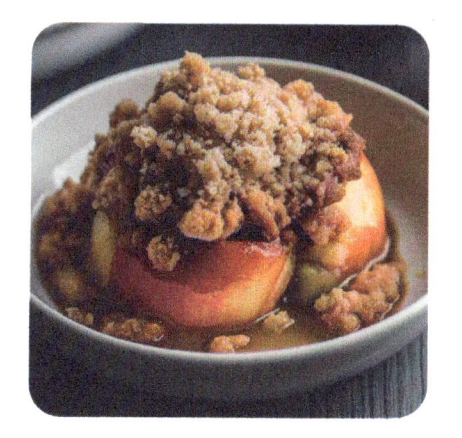

Apple Crumble

NRV (per serving):
- Calories: 220
- Protein: 3g
- Fat: 10g
- Carbohydrates: 35g
- Fiber: 6g
- Sugars: 20g

Ingredients (for 4 people):
- 4 apples, peeled and sliced
- 1 teaspoon ground cinnamon
- 1 tablespoon lemon juice
- 1/2 cup rolled oats
- 1/4 cup chopped almonds
- 2 tablespoons maple syrup
- 2 tablespoons melted coconut oil

Instructions:
1. Preheat the oven to 350°F (175°C).
2. In a bowl, mix the apples with cinnamon and lemon juice.
3. Spread the apples in a baking dish.
4. In another bowl, mix the oats, almonds, maple syrup, and melted coconut oil.
5. Sprinkle the oat mixture over the apples.
6. Bake for 30-35 minutes or until the apples are tender and the crumble is golden.
7. Let cool slightly before serving.

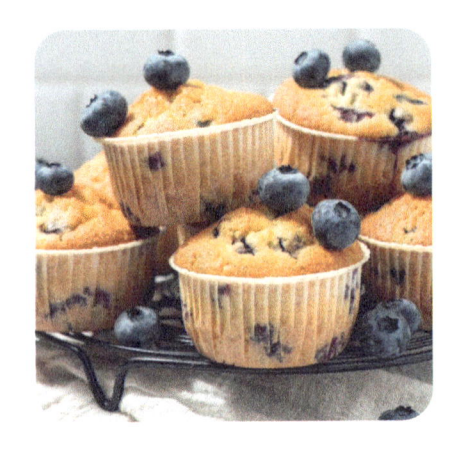

Blueberry Muffins

NRV (per muffin):
- Calories: 160
- Protein: 5g
- Fat: 6g
- Carbohydrates: 23g
- Fiber: 3g
- Sugars: 10g

Ingredients (for 12 muffins):
- 2 cups whole-wheat flour
- 1/2 cup brown sugar
- 2 teaspoons baking powder
- 1/2 teaspoon baking soda
- 1/4 teaspoon salt
- 1 cup fat-free Greek yogurt
- 2 eggs
- 1/4 cup melted coconut oil
- 1 teaspoon vanilla extract
- 1 cup fresh or frozen blueberries

Instructions:
1. Preheat the oven to 375°F (190°C) and line a muffin tin with paper liners.
2. In a large bowl, mix the flour, brown sugar, baking powder, baking soda, and salt.
3. In another bowl, whisk the yogurt, eggs, melted coconut oil, and vanilla extract.
4. Combine the wet and dry ingredients, mixing until just combined.
5. Gently fold in the blueberries.
6. Divide the batter among the muffin cups, filling them about 3/4 full.
7. Bake for 20-25 minutes or until a toothpick inserted into the center of a muffin comes out clean.
8. Let the muffins cool on a wire rack before serving.

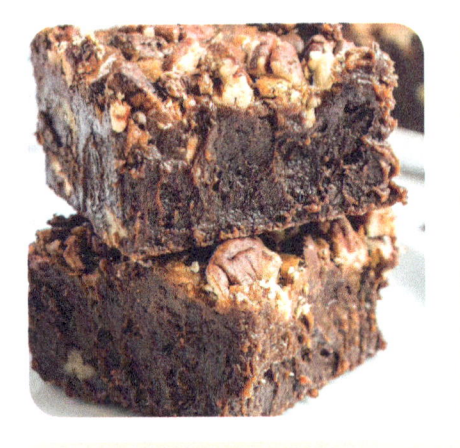

Black Bean Brownies

NRV (per brownie):
- Calories: 120
- Protein: 4g
- Fat: 6g
- Carbohydrates: 15g
- Fiber: 3g
- Sugars: 8g

Ingredients (for 16 brownies):
- 1 can black beans (15 oz), drained and rinsed
- 3 eggs
- 1/4 cup melted coconut oil
- 1/4 cup unsweetened cocoa powder
- 1/2 cup coconut sugar
- 1 teaspoon vanilla extract
- 1/2 teaspoon baking soda
- 1/4 teaspoon salt
- 1/2 cup dark chocolate chips

Instructions:
1. Preheat the oven to 350°F (175°C) and line a square baking pan with parchment paper.
2. In a blender, combine the black beans, eggs, melted coconut oil, cocoa powder, coconut sugar, vanilla extract, baking soda, and salt. Blend until smooth.
3. Pour the batter into the prepared pan and spread it evenly.
4. Sprinkle the chocolate chips on top of the batter.
5. Bake for 20-25 minutes or until a toothpick inserted into the center comes out clean.
6. Let cool completely in the pan before cutting into squares and serving.

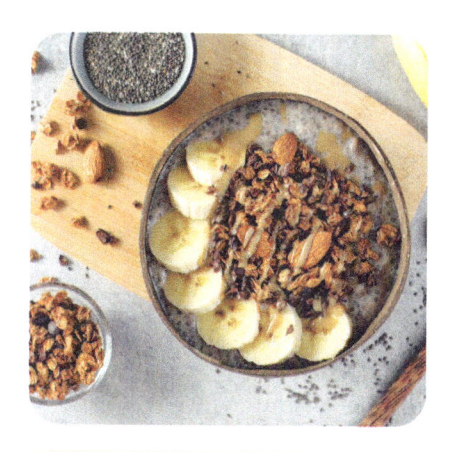

Chocolate Chia Pudding

NRV (per serving):
- Calories: 140
- Protein: 4g
- Fat: 7g
- Carbohydrates: 18g
- Fiber: 8g
- Sugars: 8g

Ingredients (for 4 people):
- 1/4 cup chia seeds
- 1 cup unsweetened almond milk
- 2 tablespoons unsweetened cocoa powder
- 2 tablespoons maple syrup
- 1 teaspoon vanilla extract
- Fresh fruit for garnish (optional)

Instructions:
1. In a bowl, mix the chia seeds, almond milk, cocoa powder, maple syrup, and vanilla extract.
2. Let sit for 10 minutes, then stir again to avoid lumps.
3. Cover the bowl and refrigerate for at least 4 hours or overnight.
4. Stir well before serving.
5. Garnish with fresh fruit if desired.

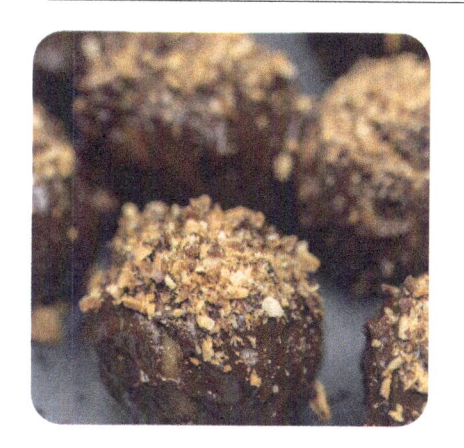

Date and Nut Truffles

NRV (per truffle):
- Calories: 80
- Protein: 2g
- Fat: 5g
- Carbohydrates: 10g
- Fiber: 2g
- Sugars: 8g

Ingredients (for 20 truffles):
- 1 cup pitted dates
- 1 cup nuts
- 1/4 cup unsweetened cocoa powder
- 1 teaspoon vanilla extract
- Pinch of salt
- Shredded coconut for garnish (optional)

Instructions:
1. In a blender or food processor, combine the dates, nuts, cocoa powder, vanilla extract, and salt. Blend until smooth.
2. Form the mixture into balls and roll them in shredded coconut if desired.
3. Place the truffles on a baking sheet lined with parchment paper.
4. Refrigerate for at least 1 hour before serving.

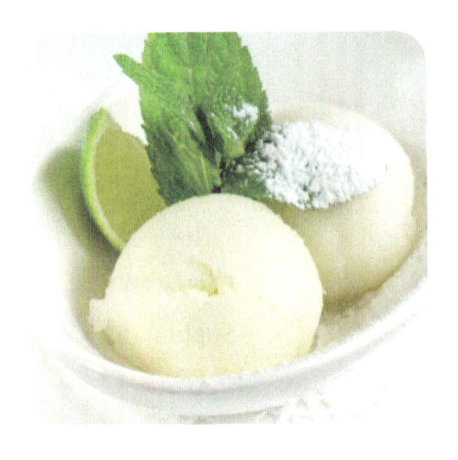

Lemon Sorbet

NRV (per serving):

- Calories: 100
- Protein: 0g
- Fat: 0g
- Carbohydrates: 27g
- Fiber: 1g
- Sugars: 20g

Ingredients (for 4 people):

- 1 cup fresh lemon juice
- 1 cup water
- 1/2 cup maple syrup
- 1 teaspoon vanilla extract
- Lemon zest for garnish (optional)

Instructions:

1. In a bowl, mix the lemon juice, water, maple syrup, and vanilla extract.
2. Pour the mixture into an ice cream maker and follow the manufacturer's instructions.
3. If you don't have an ice cream maker, pour the mixture into a baking dish and freeze, stirring every 30 minutes until the desired consistency is reached, about 2-3 hours.
4. Serve the sorbet in cups garnished with lemon zest if desired.

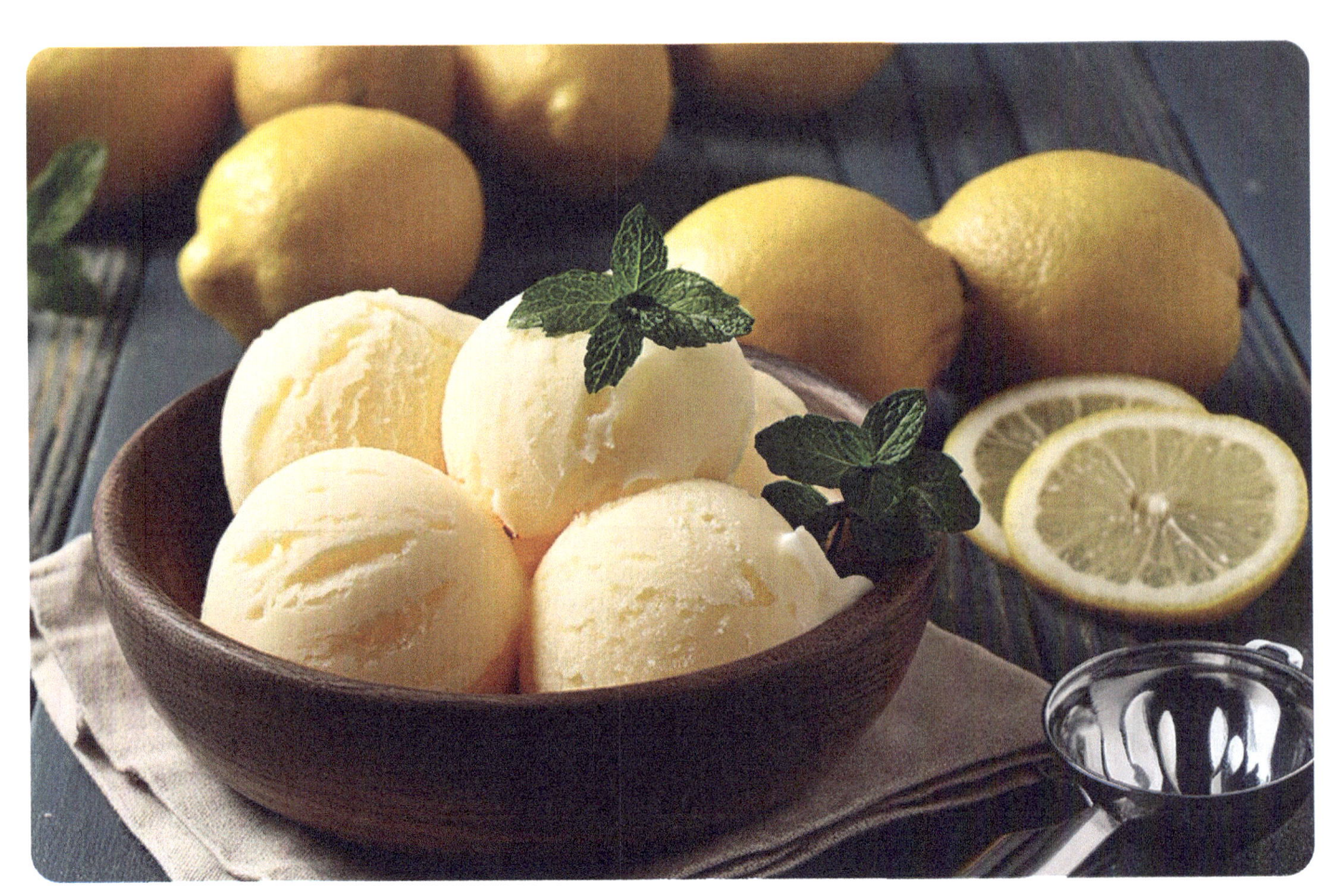

Beverages and Smoothies

Green Detox Smoothie

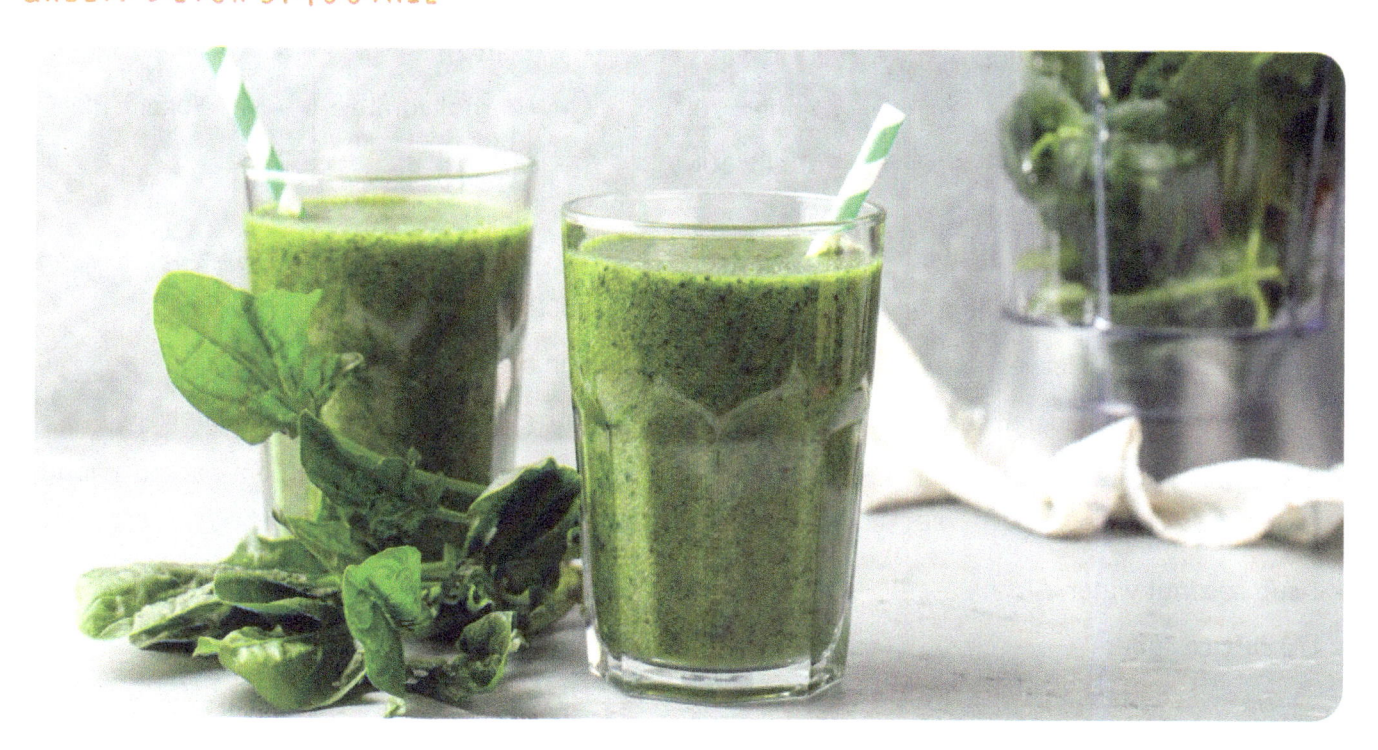

Ingredients (for 1 person):
- 1 cup fresh spinach
- 1/2 cup sliced cucumber
- 1/2 cup fresh or frozen pineapple
- 1 ripe banana
- 1/2 cup coconut water
- 1 tablespoon lemon juice
- 1/2 teaspoon fresh grated ginger

Instructions:
1. Place all ingredients in a blender.
2. Blend until smooth and consistent.
3. Pour into a glass and serve immediately.

NRV (per serving):
- Calories: 150
- Protein: 2g
- Fat: 1g
- Carbohydrates: 37g
- Fiber: 5g
- Sugars: 23g

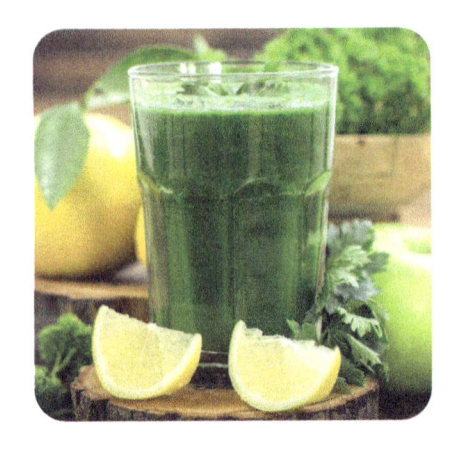

Green Apple Spinach Smoothie

NRV (per serving):
- Calories: 200
- Protein: 10g
- Fat: 2g
- Carbohydrates: 38g
- Fiber: 5g
- Sugars: 20g

Ingredients (for 2 servings):
- 1 green apple, cored and chopped
- 1 cup fresh spinach leaves
- 1/2 cucumber, peeled and chopped
- 1/2 lemon, juiced
- 1 tablespoon chia seeds
- 1 cup coconut water
- 1/2 cup ice cubes

Instructions:
1. Place all the ingredients into a blender.
2. Blend on high until smooth and creamy.
3. Pour into glasses and serve immediately.
4. Enjoy your refreshing and nutrient-packed smoothie.

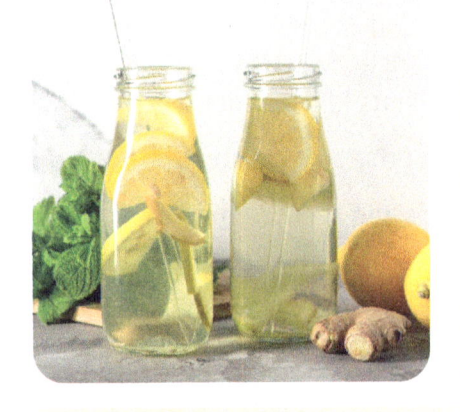

Lemon Ginger Detox Water

NRV (per serving):
- Calories: 5
- Protein: 0g
- Fat: 0g
- Carbohydrates: 1g
- Fiber: 0g
- Sugars: 0g

Ingredients (for 4 people):
- 1 liter of water
- 1 lemon, sliced
- 1 inch fresh ginger, sliced
- 1/4 cup fresh mint leaves

Instructions:
1. In a pitcher, combine the water, lemon slices, ginger, and mint leaves.
2. Stir well and let it sit in the refrigerator for at least 1 hour before serving.
3. Serve the detox water chilled.

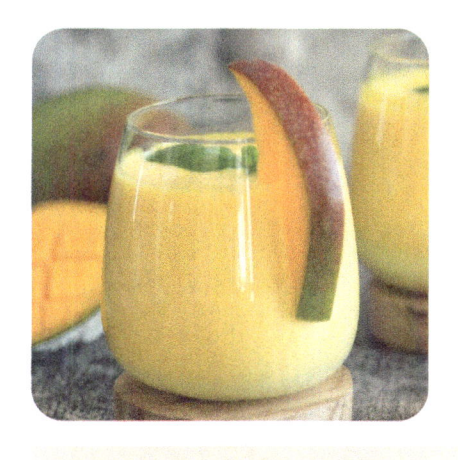

Mango Turmeric Smoothie

NRV (per serving):
- Calories: 180
- Protein: 2g
- Fat: 4g
- Carbohydrates: 38g
- Fiber: 4g
- Sugars: 32g

Ingredients (for 1 person):
- 1 cup fresh or frozen mango
- 1 ripe banana
- 1/2 cup light coconut milk
- 1/2 teaspoon turmeric powder
- 1/2 teaspoon lemon juice

Instructions:
1. Place the mango, banana, coconut milk, turmeric, and lemon juice in a blender.
2. Blend until smooth and consistent.
3. Pour into a glass and serve immediately.

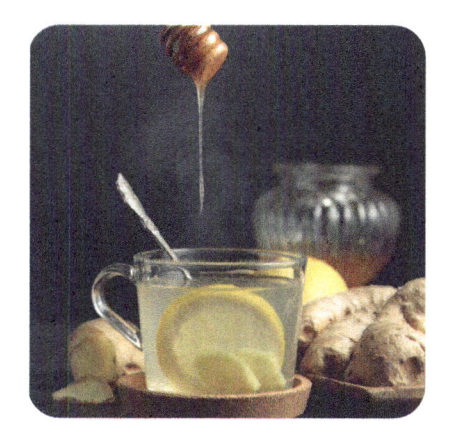

Lemon Ginger Tea

NRV (per serving):
- Calories: 20
- Protein: 0g
- Fat: 0g
- Carbohydrates: 6g
- Fiber: 0g
- Sugars: 5g

Ingredients (for 2 people):
- 2 cups water
- 1 inch fresh ginger, sliced
- Juice of 1 lemon
- 1 tablespoon honey (optional)

Instructions:
1. Bring the water to a boil in a saucepan.
2. Add the sliced ginger and reduce the heat. Let it simmer for 10 minutes.
3. Remove from heat and add the lemon juice and honey if desired.
4. Pour the tea into cups and serve warm.

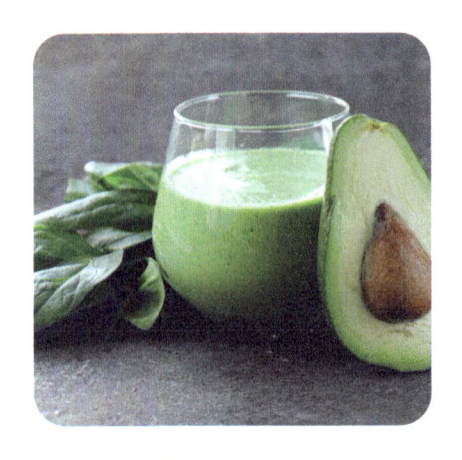

Avocado Spinach Smoothie

NRV (per serving):
- Calories: 220
- Protein: 3g
- Fat: 11g
- Carbohydrates: 30g
- Fiber: 7g
- Sugars: 12g

Ingredients (for 1 person):
- 1/2 ripe avocado
- 1 cup fresh spinach
- 1 ripe banana
- 1 cup unsweetened almond milk
- 1 teaspoon honey (optional)

Instructions:
5. Place the avocado, spinach, banana, and almond milk in a blender.
6. Blend until smooth and consistent.
7. Add honey if desired and blend again.
8. Pour into a glass and serve immediately.

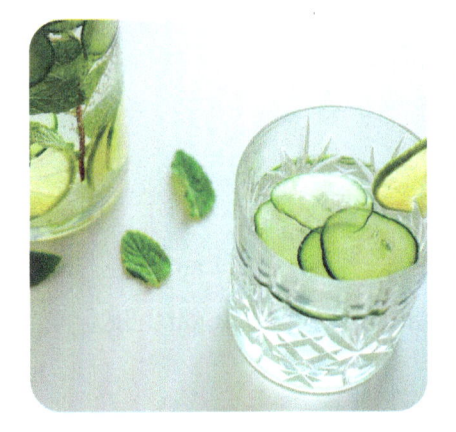

Cucumber Mint Water

NRV (per serving):
- Calories: 5
- Protein: 0g
- Fat: 0g
- Carbohydrates: 1g
- Fiber: 0g
- Sugars: 0g

Ingredients (for 4 people):
- 1 liter of water
- 1 cucumber, sliced
- 1/4 cup fresh mint leaves
- Juice of 1 lime

Instructions:
1. In a pitcher, combine the water, cucumber slices, mint leaves, and lime juice.
2. Stir well and let it sit in the refrigerator for at least 1 hour before serving.
3. Serve the water chilled.

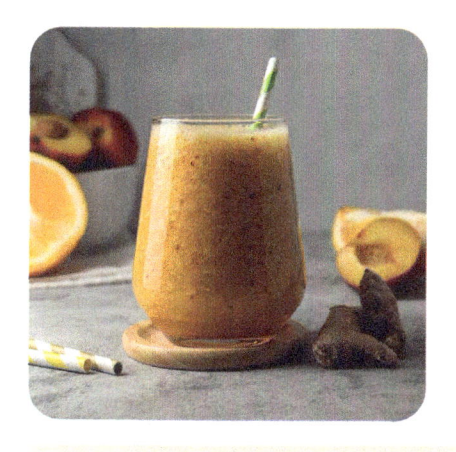

Peach Ginger Smoothie

NRV (per serving):
- Calories: 180
- Protein: 8g
- Fat: 1g
- Carbohydrates: 36g
- Fiber: 4g
- Sugars: 28g

Ingredients (for 1 person):
- 1 cup fresh or frozen peaches
- 1 ripe banana
- 1/2 cup fat-free Greek yogurt
- 1/2 cup orange juice
- 1/2 teaspoon fresh grated ginger

Instructions:
1. Place the peaches, banana, Greek yogurt, orange juice, and ginger in a blender.
2. Blend until smooth and consistent.
3. Pour into a glass and serve immediately.

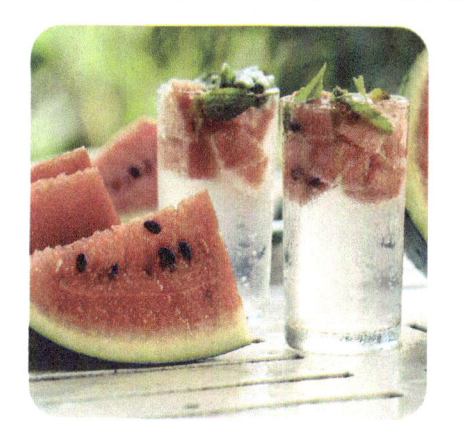

Watermelon Mint Water

NRV (per serving):
- Calories: 10
- Protein: 0g
- Fat: 0g
- Carbohydrates: 2g
- Fiber: 0g
- Sugars: 2g

Ingredients (for 4 people):
- 1 liter of water
- 2 cups watermelon, cubed
- 1/4 cup fresh mint leaves

Instructions:
1. In a pitcher, combine the water, watermelon cubes, and mint leaves.
2. Stir well and let it sit in the refrigerator for at least 1 hour before serving.
3. Serve the water chilled.

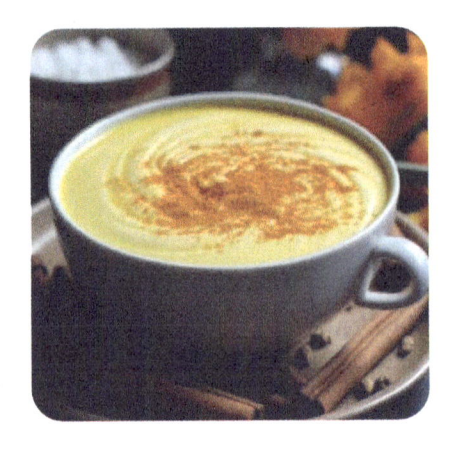

Golden Milk

NRV (per serving):
- Calories: 70
- Protein: 1g
- Fat: 3g
- Carbohydrates: 10g
- Fiber: 2g
- Sugars: 7g

Ingredients (for 2 people):
- 2 cups unsweetened almond milk
- 1 teaspoon turmeric powder
- 1/2 teaspoon cinnamon powder
- 1/4 teaspoon ginger powder
- 1 tablespoon honey (optional)
- Pinch of black pepper

Instructions:
1. In a saucepan, heat the almond milk over medium heat.
2. Add the turmeric, cinnamon, ginger, and black pepper.
3. Stir well and cook for 5 minutes without boiling.
4. Add honey if desired and stir until dissolved.
5. Pour into cups and serve warm.

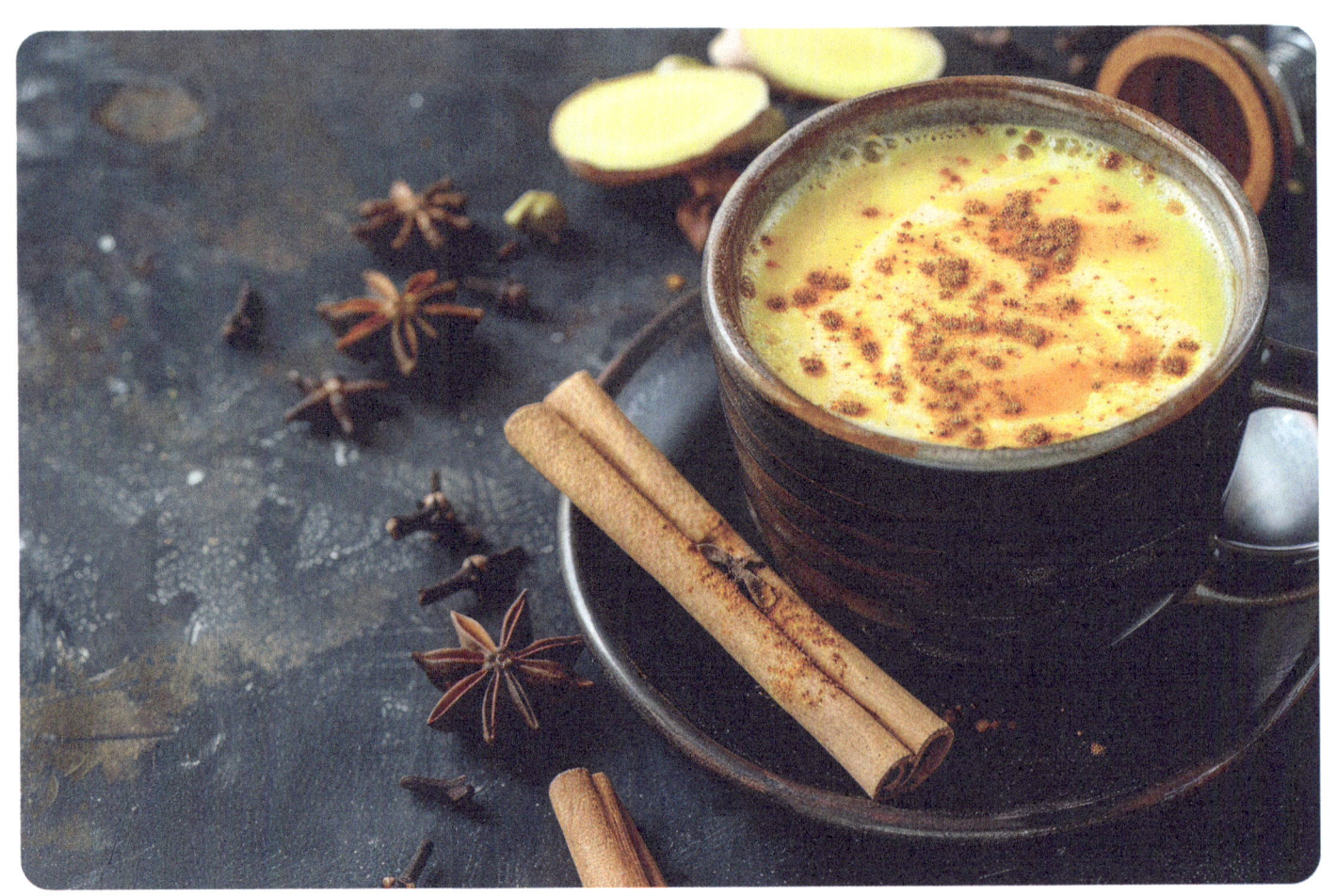

28-Day Meal Plan

As promised, here is the 28-day meal plan. Four complete weeks to help you organize your meals and make the most of the recipes contained in the previous chapter. This plan is not rigid and can be adjusted to your needs and the ingredients available in your pantry. Feel free to adapt it as necessary.

Week 1

Day 1:
- **Breakfast:** Banana Oat Pancakes
- **Lunch:** Grilled Chicken Salad
- **Dinner:** Baked Salmon with Asparagus
- **Snack:** Hummus with Crudités

Day 2:
- **Breakfast:** Egg and Vegetable Muffins
- **Lunch:** Turkey and Vegetable Wrap
- **Dinner:** Grilled Chicken with Mixed Vegetables
- **Snack:** Greek Yogurt with Honey and Nuts

Day 3:
- **Breakfast:** Greek Yogurt and Muesli Parfait
- **Lunch:** Quinoa Salad with Chickpeas and Vegetables
- **Dinner:** Vegetable Soup with Quinoa
- **Snack:** Kale Chips

Day 4:
- **Breakfast:** Avocado Toast with Poached Eggs
- **Lunch:** Black Bean and Corn Salad
- **Dinner:** Coconut Curry Chicken
- **Snack:** Green Smoothie

Day 5:
- **Breakfast:** Quinoa Porridge with Berries
- **Lunch:** Buddha Bowl with Tofu and Vegetables
- **Dinner:** Lemon Caper Cod Fillets
- **Snack:** Fruit Skewers

Day 6:
- **Breakfast:** Berry Smoothie Bowl
- **Lunch:** Spinach Salad with Salmon and Avocado
- **Dinner:** Grilled Tofu with Peanut Sauce
- **Snack:** Guacamole with Vegetable Sticks

Day 7:
- **Breakfast:** Whole Wheat Toast with Ricotta and Fruit
- **Lunch:** Lentil and Vegetable Soup
- **Dinner:** Lemon Caper Chicken
- **Snack:** Deviled Eggs

Week 2

Day 8:
- **Breakfast:** Scrambled Eggs with Avocado and Tomato
- **Lunch:** Tuna Salad with Green Beans and Potatoes
- **Dinner:** Zucchini Noodles with Cherry Tomatoes and Basil
- **Snack:** Strawberry Banana Smoothie

Day 9:
- **Breakfast:** Chia Pudding with Almond Milk and Fruit
- **Lunch:** Turkey and Avocado Wrap
- **Dinner:** Mushroom Risotto
- **Snack:** Steamed Edamame with Sea Salt

Day 10:
- **Breakfast:** Asparagus and Feta Frittata
- **Lunch:** Sesame Chicken with Zucchini
- **Dinner:** Chickpea and Tuna Salad
- **Snack:** Blueberry Oat Bars

Day 11:
- **Breakfast:** Blueberry Spinach Smoothie
- **Lunch:** Grilled Pork Tenderloin with Vegetables
- **Dinner:** Chicken and Vegetable Soup
- **Snack:** Mixed Fruit with Greek Yogurt

Day 12:
- **Breakfast:** Banana Oat Pancakes
- **Lunch:** Grilled Chicken Salad
- **Dinner:** Spinach and Mushroom Frittata
- **Snack:** Melon Wrapped in Prosciutto

Day 13:
- **Breakfast:** Egg and Vegetable Muffins
- **Lunch:** Turkey and Vegetable Wrap
- **Dinner:** Polenta with Mushrooms and Spinach
- **Snack:** Cucumber Sticks with Yogurt Dip

Day 14:
- **Breakfast:** Greek Yogurt and Muesli Parfait
- **Lunch:** Quinoa Salad with Chickpeas and Vegetables
- **Dinner:** Baked Turkey Meatballs with Tomato Sauce
- **Snack:** Hummus with Crudités

Week 3

Day 15:
- **Breakfast:** Avocado Toast with Poached Eggs
- **Lunch:** Black Bean and Corn Salad
- **Dinner:** Baked Salmon with Asparagus
- **Snack:** Greek Yogurt with Honey and Nuts

Day 16:
- **Breakfast:** Quinoa Porridge with Berries
- **Lunch:** Buddha Bowl with Tofu and Vegetables
- **Dinner:** Grilled Chicken with Mixed Vegetables
- **Snack:** Kale Chips

Day 17:
- **Breakfast:** Berry Smoothie Bowl
- **Lunch:** Spinach Salad with Salmon and Avocado
- **Dinner:** Vegetable Soup with Quinoa
- **Snack:** Green Smoothie

Day 18:
- **Breakfast:** Whole Wheat Toast with Ricotta and Fruit

- **Lunch:** Lentil and Vegetable Soup
- **Dinner:** Coconut Curry Chicken
- **Snack:** Fruit Skewers

Day 19:
- **Breakfast:** Scrambled Eggs with Avocado and Tomato
- **Lunch:** Tuna Salad with Green Beans and Potatoes
- **Dinner:** Lemon Caper Cod Fillets
- **Snack:** Guacamole with Vegetable Sticks

Day 20:
- **Breakfast:** Chia Pudding with Almond Milk and Fruit
- **Lunch:** Turkey and Avocado Wrap
- **Dinner:** Grilled Tofu with Peanut Sauce
- **Snack:** Deviled Eggs

Day 21:
- **Breakfast:** Asparagus and Feta Frittata
- **Lunch:** Sesame Chicken with Zucchini
- **Dinner:** Zucchini Noodles with Cherry Tomatoes and Basil
- **Snack:** Strawberry Banana Smoothie

Week 4

Day 22:
- **Breakfast:** Blueberry Spinach Smoothie
- **Lunch:** Grilled Pork Tenderloin with Vegetables
- **Dinner:** Mushroom Risotto
- **Snack:** Steamed Edamame with Sea Salt

Day 23:
- **Breakfast:** Banana Oat Pancakes
- **Lunch:** Grilled Chicken Salad
- **Dinner:** Chickpea and Tuna Salad
- **Snack:** Blueberry Oat Bars

Day 24:
- **Breakfast:** Egg and Vegetable Muffins
- **Lunch:** Turkey and Vegetable Wrap
- **Dinner:** Chicken and Vegetable Soup
- **Snack:** Mixed Fruit with Greek Yogurt

Day 25:
- **Breakfast:** Greek Yogurt and Muesli Parfait
- **Lunch:** Quinoa Salad with Chickpeas and Vegetables
- **Dinner:** Polenta with Mushrooms and Spinach
- **Snack:** Melon Wrapped in Prosciutto

Day 26:
- **Breakfast:** Avocado Toast with Poached Eggs
- **Lunch:** Black Bean and Corn Salad
- **Dinner:** Baked Turkey Meatballs with Tomato Sauce
- **Snack:** Cucumber Sticks with Yogurt Dip

Day 27:
- **Breakfast:** Quinoa Porridge with Berries
- **Lunch:** Buddha Bowl with Tofu and Vegetables
- **Dinner:** Baked Salmon with Asparagus
- **Snack:** Hummus with Crudités

Day 28:
- **Breakfast:** Berry Smoothie Bowl
- **Lunch:** Spinach Salad with Salmon and Avocado
- **Dinner:** Grilled Chicken with Mixed Vegetables
- **Snack:** Greek Yogurt with Honey and Nuts

Measurement Conversions

Measurement Conversion Table

American Measure	Metric System Equivalent
1 cup	240 ml
1/2 cup	120 ml
1/3 cup	80 ml
1/4 cup	60 ml
1 tablespoon	15 ml
1 teaspoon	5 ml
1/2 teaspoon	2.5 ml
1/4 teaspoon	1.25 ml
1 oz (ounce)	28 g
1 lb (pound)	454 g
1 pint	473 ml
1 quart	946 ml
1 gallon	3.78 liters

Oven Temperature Conversion

Fahrenheit (°F)	Celsius (°C)
250°F	120°C
300°F	150°C
350°F	175°C
375°F	190°C
400°F	200°C
425°F	220°C
450°F	230°C
475°F	245°C
500°F	260°C

Common Ingredient Conversions

Ingredient	American Measure	Metric System Equivalent
Flour	1 cup	120 g
Sugar	1 cup	200 g
Powdered Sugar	1 cup	120 g
Butter	1 tablespoon	14 g
Rice	1 cup	185 g
Oats	1 cup	90 g
Chopped Almonds/Walnuts	1 cup	120 g
Honey	1 cup	340 g
Milk	1 cup	240 ml
Yogurt	1 cup	245 g

Conclusion

We have reached the end of the "0 Point Weight Loss Cookbook." This culinary journey has been designed to offer you delicious, nutritious, and, above all, "0 point" recipes. My hope is that you have found inspiration and motivation to embrace a healthier and more balanced lifestyle without sacrificing the taste and pleasure of eating.

A New Beginning

Adopting a "0 point" diet does not mean depriving yourself, but rather making conscious choices that nourish both body and mind. The recipes contained in this book demonstrate that it is possible to enjoy flavorful and satisfying dishes while maintaining control over your weight and overall well-being.

Variety is Key

Variety is one of the fundamental aspects of maintaining a balanced and sustainable diet. The recipes for breakfasts, lunches, dinners, snacks, and desserts offer a wide range of options that you can combine and adapt to your personal preferences. Don't hesitate to experiment and make adjustments to make each dish perfect for you.

Planning and Preparation

As we saw in the 28-day meal plan, planning is essential for long-term success. Preparing meals in advance, making a targeted shopping list, and organizing your time in the kitchen can make a big difference. Remember that preparation is half the battle!

Stay Motivated

The journey to a healthier life can present challenges, but don't let yourself get discouraged. Stay motivated by keeping your goals in mind and celebrating your successes, no matter how big or small. The key is consistency and dedication.

A Special Thank You

Thank you for choosing the "0 Point Weight Loss Cookbook." I hope that the recipes and tips contained in these pages have inspired and helped you on your wellness journey. Keep exploring, cooking, and enjoying every moment of this journey towards a healthier and happier life.

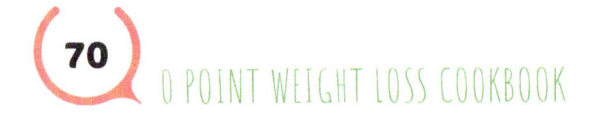

If you enjoyed the book, I would be grateful if you left me an honest review on Amazon. I would really appreciate it!

Share Your Success

Finally, don't forget to share your success and experiences with friends and family. Cooking together and exchanging recipes can be a wonderful way to strengthen bonds and motivate each other.

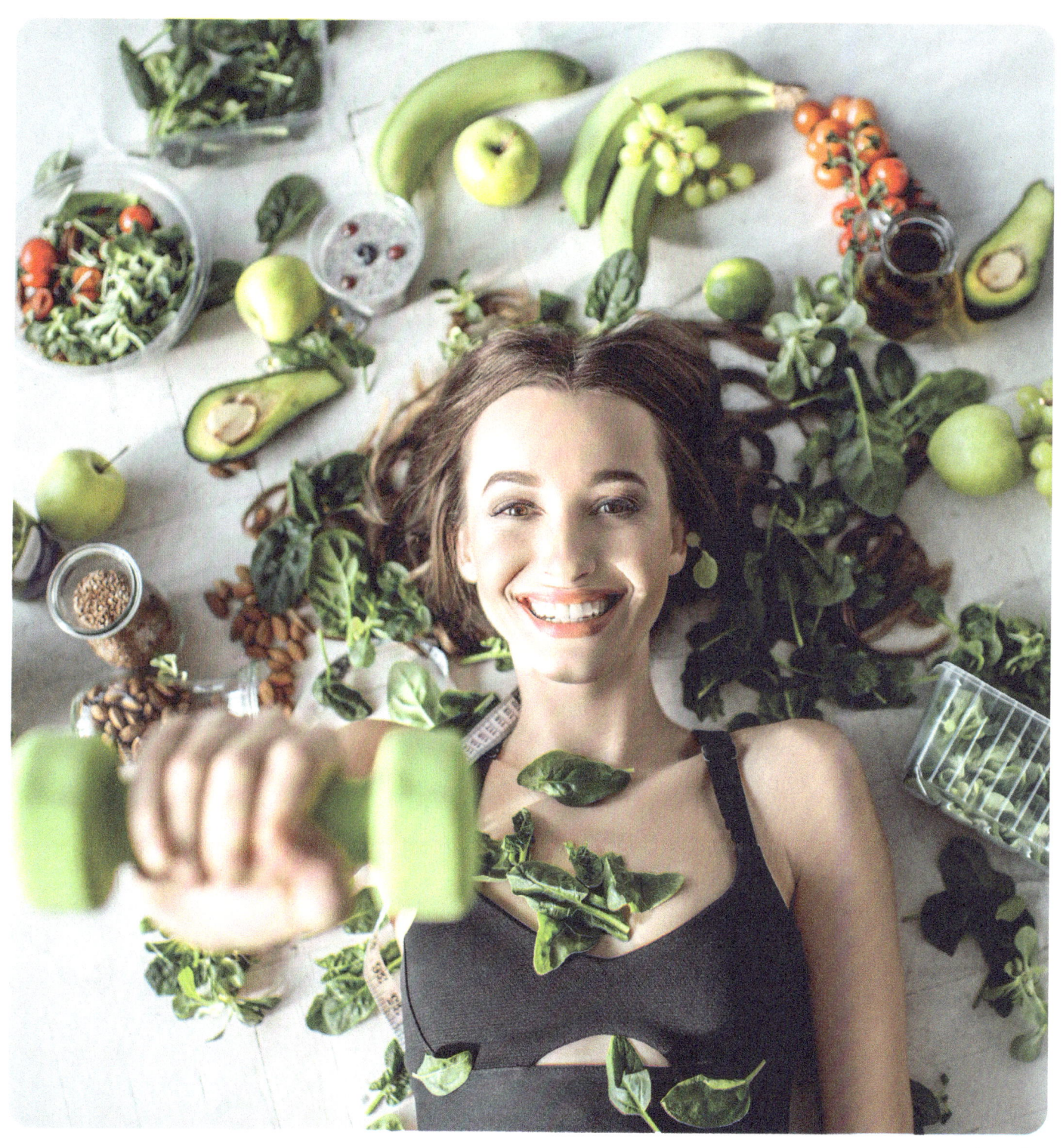

Recipe Index

Apple Cinnamon Oatmeal	22
Apple Crumble	55
Asparagus and Feta Frittata	28
Avocado Chocolate Mousse	53
Avocado Spinach Smoothie	62
Avocado Toast with Poached Eggs	25
Baked Salmon with Asparagus	45
Baked Turkey Meatballs with Tomato Sauce	48
Banana Oat Pancakes	24
Banana Peanut Butter Ice Cream	54
Barley Salad with Roasted Vegetables	35
Berry Cheesecake	55
Berry Smoothie Bowl	26
Black Bean and Corn Salad	33
Black Bean Brownies	56
Blueberry Muffins	56
Blueberry Oat Bars	42
Blueberry Spinach Smoothie	42
Brown Rice with Curry Vegetables	33
Buddha Bowl with Tofu and Vegetable	32
Cereal and Nut Bars	43
Chia Pudding with Almond Milk and Fruit	28
Chicken and Vegetable Soup	51
Chickpea and Tuna Salad	49
Chocolate Chia Pudding	57
Coconut Curry Chicken	34
Coconut Panna Cotta	54
Cucumber Mint Water	62
Cucumber Sticks with Yogurt Dip	44
Date and Nut Truffles	57
Deviled Eggs	40
Egg and Vegetable Muffins	24
Egg White Omelette with Spinach and Tomatoes	22
Fish Tacos with Avocado Sauce	31
Fruit Skewers	39
Golden Milk	64
Greek Yogurt and Muesli Parfait	24
Greek Yogurt with Fruit and Nuts	23
Greek Yogurt with Honey and Nuts	38
Green Apple Spinach Smoothie	60
Green Detox Smoothie	59
Green Smoothie	39

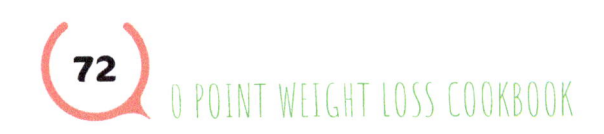

Grilled Chicken Salad	29
Grilled Chicken with Mixed Vegetables	46
Grilled Pork Tenderloin with Vegetables	51
Grilled Tofu with Peanut Sauce	47
Guacamole with Vegetable Sticks	40
Hummus with Crudités	37
Kale and Apple Salad	36
Kale Chips	38
Lemon Caper Chicken	50
Lemon Caper Cod Fillets	48
Lemon Ginger Detox Water	60
Lemon Ginger Tea	61
Lemon Sorbet	58
Lentil and Vegetable Soup	30
Mango Turmeric Smoothie	61
Melon Wrapped in Prosciutto	44
Mixed Fruit with Greek Yogurt	43
Mushroom Risotto	49
Peach Ginger Smoothie	63
Polenta with Mushrooms and Spinach	52
Quinoa Porridge with Berries	26
Quinoa Salad with Chickpeas and Vegetables	31
Scrambled Eggs with Avocado and Tomato	27
Sesame Chicken with Zucchini	50
Spinach and Berry Smoothie	21
Spinach and Mushroom Frittata	52
Spinach Salad with Salmon and Avocado	32
Steamed Edamame with Sea Salt	41
Strawberry Banana Smoothie	41
Tomato Basil Soup	36
Tuna Salad with Green Beans and Potatoes	34
Turkey and Avocado Wrap	35
Turkey and Vegetable Wrap	30
Vegetable Frittata	23
Vegetable Soup with Quinoa	46
Watermelon Mint Water	63
Whole Wheat Toast with Ricotta and Fruit	27
Zucchini Noodles with Cherry Tomatoes and Basil	47

BONUS

Get your exclusive BONUS now!

A 56-page ebook, created directly by me, containing 6 bonus chapters to expand and deepen your knowledge on the **"ZERO POINT DIET"**!

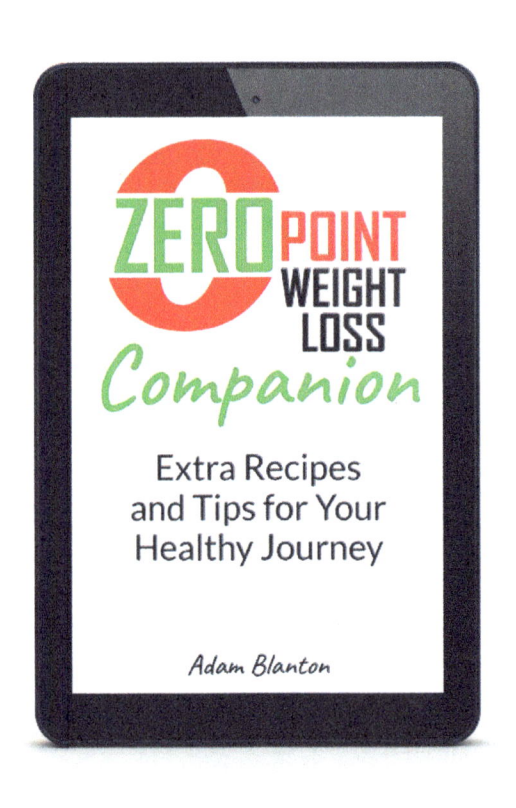

Scan the QR CODE to download the BONUS reserved for you!

NOTES

Notes

Notes

Notes

Notes

Made in the USA
Coppell, TX
23 April 2025